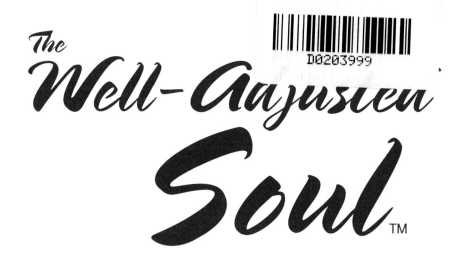

The Well-Adjusted Soul™

FEEL-GOOD STORIES FROM THE HEART OF CHIROPRACTIC

FABRIZIO MANCINI, DC
CO-AUTHOR, CHICKEN SOUP FOR THE CHIROPRACTIC SOUL

GILLES A. LAMARCHE, DC
CO-AUTHOR, CHIROPRACTIC FROM THE HEART

DONALD M. DIBLE, MS
SERIES EDITOR

PARKER
SEMINARS

Dallas, Texas

VOLUME 1

Published by Parker College of Chiropractic
d/b/a Parker Seminars

Copyright © 2010 Parker College of Chiropractic
d/b/a Parker Seminars

Permissions Acknowledgments appear on page 316.

Cataloging-in-Publication Data is on file with the Library of Congress

Library of Congress Control Number: 2010936595

ISBN: 978-0-615-38960-8

Parker Seminars
Rights and Permissions Department
2500 Walnut Hill Lane
Suite S-212
Dallas, Texas 75229

In the spirit of creating a healthier lifestyle through Chiropractic care, a portion of the proceeds will go toward a fund for the advancement of Chiropractic education, research, and public relations. If you feel inspired to join us in this cause of bringing Chiropractic to the ones you love with your contributions or donations, please contact us at www.parkerseminars.com or 888.772.5867. Your contributions truly will make a difference.

These stories hopefully provide general education, inspiration, and nourishment for your soul. However, every individual is unique as is their health. You deserve and need the careful thought and individual attention of your own doctor to determine the condition of your health and to decide how you should respond to, or treat, any disease or condition that you may have. No matter how entertaining and heartwarming this book may be, it cannot replace a doctor-patient relationship or provide a diagnosis, prescription, or recommendation for you or your condition.

Cover by Lily Xu Designs, Pleasanton, California

Interior design and formatting by DMD House, Murrieta, California
www.dmdhousebooks.com

Cartoons reprinted by arrangement with
Finkstrom Licensing International http://finkstrom.com

Contents

4. Birth Trauma

5. Pediatric Wellness

6. Coping with Life's Challenges

7. Recovering Sight and Hearing

8. Patient Comeback Stories

9. I Got My Life Back!

10. Surgery? Just Say No!

11. Chiropractic and Sports

12. Chiropractic Tributes

13. The Golden Years

14. A Chiropractic Menagerie

Introduction

Decades before the 150-million-copies-sold Chicken Soup for the Soul® phenomenon came into being—back when I was a "starving student," Chiropractic entered my life. At the time, I was an aspiring teacher at the University of Massachusetts Amherst, Graduate School of Education; and I had suffered with chronic neck and upper-shoulder pain for years. When I complained to a wiser-than-me classmate about my problem, he suggested that I consider Chiropractic—a non-invasive, pill-free, non-surgical healthcare option. "What have I got to lose? That sounds like a no-brainer!" I thought to myself. My classmate then provided me with a referral to his own doctor.

The chiropractor discovered during his initial exam that my left leg was shorter than the right leg. This imbalance was throwing my hips out of whack. In turn, that threw the vertebrae in my spine out of alignment—causing what chiropractors call "subluxations." It was multiple subluxations—misaligned vertebrae pinching the nerves at various places along my spine—that were causing the pain.

The chiropractor prescribed an orthotic, a special lift that was placed in my left shoe to even out my leg length. Between the orthotic and a series of regular adjustments, my body function improved and my shoulder and neck pain completely vanished. There was also a surprise, added benefit: I started sleeping more soundly! From that point on, I accepted the fact that having a well-adjusted spine was important to my pain-free health and happiness. I also understood that in normal life, my body is going to have to deal with occasional physical and emotional stresses that can pull-push my spine out of alignment and negatively affect my nervous system. That's why I'm committed to regular Chiropractic care.

Some years after graduating from UMass Amherst, I accepted a position with a large seminar training organization and moved to Los Angeles. The company's offices were located on the second floor of a building directly above a large Chiropractic clinic. Many of our students were chiropractors—including most of the doctors on the clinic staff. Since I had already come to associate wellbeing with regular Chiropractic care, and because the clinic was so close to my work, I got adjusted three-to-four times a week—and felt GREAT! Sometimes after an adjustment, I'd experience an almost euphoric glow as my body's energy would rush to places where, previously, it had been blocked.

A big thing that locked me into loving Chiropractic was when my third son was born. He couldn't nurse properly. Although he would suck on your little finger if you stuck it in his mouth, the stimulus of his mother's soft breast didn't trigger his sucking reflex. Fearing that he might have a major neurological disorder, my wife and I took him to a pediatrician who subsequently referred us to a neurologist. Our son's condition did not improve.

Then, I started thinking about Chiropractic. It occurred to me that our infant might have suffered birth trauma with a resulting misalignment of his spine. So I said to my wife, "Honey, let's go see a chiropractor." Almost immediately after our son's first adjustment, he started nursing just like any healthy baby. Of course, we had him adjusted regularly for some time after that.

When the children got older, we'd take them with us on vacation to Hawaii. During one trip, it was only a few days after we arrived when I was body surfing alone in high waves shortly after a storm had passed. I didn't notice that the weather-wise local residents weren't in the water. I got totally spun around, kicked up, and bent by the heavy surf. I could hear the crunching as tissues in my neck got stretched when a rogue wave threw me down onto the sandy beach; I hoped I hadn't broken any vertebrae. Moments later, my neck got warm and I was afraid to try and move it for fear I wouldn't be able to. I wasted no time getting out of the water and looking up a local chiropractor. He adjusted me several times before our family returned to the mainland. In other words, I see chiropractors for regular maintenance and assessments and whenever I experience trauma—regardless of where I am. Recently, I was recommending Chiropractic to a friend when he asked how many different practitioners I had seen in my life. It took me a few minutes to consider my answer: more than thirty!

Once the Chicken Soup books took off, and for a period of five years after that, I had a chiropractor visit our home once a week to adjust the whole family—a luxury I was finally able to afford and could easily justify on health grounds. Another result of the Chicken Soup success has been a radical increase in my number of speaking engagements—more than 100 convention talks and workshops annually. Many of these require international travel where I might spend as much as twenty hours—each way—sitting in airline seats for a single presentation. The rigors of trips like that often lock me up! You can be sure a special visit to the chiropractor's office for an adjustment is high on my priority list once I return from long trips like these.

Another outcome associated with the success of Chicken Soup for the Soul® is the size of the convention audiences I'm privileged to keynote. On one occasion, I addressed 7,000 delegates at the Scottrade Arena in St. Louis. Following my presentation, I autographed books almost nonstop from 5:00pm to midnight! (To date, I'm certain I've signed more than 100,000 books!) Given the wear and tear that autograph marathons like this cause on my right wrist, it shouldn't surprise you that I'm occasionally bothered with carpal tunnel syndrome. As the Ghostbusters' song asks, "Who ya' gonna' call?" For carpal tunnel relief—and a whole lot more, I call my chiropractor!

That brings me to the reason why I accepted the invitation of Parker Seminars to write the Introduction for this book. As you can see from my own life-experiences, my family and I have benefitted enormously from the health-giving wonders of Chiropractic. The book you now hold in your hands contains 75 stories and testimonials attesting to the effectiveness of this remarkable healing art. If you have been reluctant to personally try the benefits of Chiropractic, or if you know someone whose health you believe could be improved with this care, I urge you to read this book and then pass it on. The stories and testimonials in *The Well-Adjusted Soul* make a powerful statement that deserves to be shared far and wide. You have my word on that!

Jack Canfield
Co-creator of Chicken Soup for the Soul®
Co-author of *The Success Principles:*
How to Get from Where You Are to Where You Want to Be

Foreword

My name is Dr. James Chestnut, and I have been asked to write a Foreword for this book. At first I was very hesitant; as a scientist I can be very left-brain biased, and I am not often attracted to—or moved by—emotional, "feel-good stories."

I am, however, emotionally moved by injustice, prejudice, and dogma. I have no tolerance for such things, and they elicit very strong, even visceral, reactions from me. I am also very highly emotional about the issues of promoting health and alleviating human suffering. So, when prejudice and dogma are involved in an injustice that causes human suffering—or interferes with the ability to promote health—I become morally outraged; I become inspired to take action.

I chose to contribute to this book for one reason only; because I feel morally obligated to take any opportunity that presents itself to alleviate the prejudice and dogma that has prevented so many from being helped by Chiropractic. Ignorance I can tolerate— I am ignorant about many things.

Prejudice I cannot tolerate. Prejudice is condemnation without investigation. Prejudice is dangerous; it is unethical; it is evil. Dogma is *prejudice* disguised as *educated opinion*; it is the basis of cult. It is insidious; it is cancerous; it is repugnant.

Let me briefly introduce myself. By training, I am a teacher, a scientist, and a chiropractor—I have a bachelor's degree in Education, a Masters Degree in Science (Physiology), and I am a Doctor of Chiropractic. In total, I spent 14 years in post-secondary education and have spent more than 25 years reading scientific research every day. I am passionate—some would say obsessive—about understanding how the human body works, why humans get sick, and discovering the most evidence-based ways to get and keep humans well.

I *became* a chiropractor because of a personal experience that is really only extraordinary if you are not familiar with Chiropractic.

As a young man, I was injured while playing rugby—a vigorous contact sport and one of the world's oldest forms of "football"— while attending college in Canada. As a scholarship athlete, I was given access to the very best of medical care. I was "promoted" to the front of all the medical waiting lists. Nevertheless, I did not find anyone who could properly diagnose or correct my problem. I saw several medical doctors including a neurologist—no relief! I tried physiotherapy—no relief! I tried acupuncture—no relief! I tried massage—you guessed it: No Relief! Nothing Was Working!

For an entire year, I trusted the guidance of those charged with providing traditional medical care to help me. During those twelve months, I moved robot-like from one medical referral to the next. Finally, after a year of pain, disability, frustration, and even *depression*—from not being able to play rugby without extreme pain, I decided to take charge of my own health options. I did this against the advice of the people in whom I had put my trust and faith. *I went to see a chiropractor!* The results were so extraordinary that I declined my acceptance to pursue a PhD and chose, instead, to become a Doctor of Chiropractic.

As you might imagine, the reaction to this news was not over-whelmingly positive. My father has a PhD; the people who wrote letters of recommendation for me to get accepted into a PhD program were PhDs; and one of my advisors for my master's thesis was an MD. None of them were exactly thrilled with my deci-sion. All but one—including members of my own family—had some form of negative bias against Chiropractic ranging from *dismissive arrogance* to outright *dogmatic prejudice!*

The one PhD who *had* done some investigation into Chiropractic was actually *very positive about the profession!* He was also well aware of the prejudice against it. In fact, he had seen this prejudice first hand when asked to participate on a committee at the university to discuss whether or not to include a Chiropractic program as part of the curriculum. I will always be grateful for this man's candor; and I will always remember the look of sadness on his face when he discussed anti-Chiropractic *prejudice* and *dogma* rather than *scientific resistance* to Chiropractic. He confided in me that none of his academic colleagues that were opposed to Chiropractic had ever offered one bit of *scientific evidence* to support their viewpoint—it was all based on *prejudice* and *dogma.*

Perhaps even more shocking to me was that the medical doctor whom I had seen on and off for more than a year due to my devastating injury had not only advised against even *trying* Chiropractic—he said it was dangerous and did not work—but showed not a single shred of joy on my behalf when I shared the news that I had been helped so dramatically.

At that point I realized two things. First, I understood that my medical doctor was not in the least bit interested in hearing about how a chiropractor had helped me. To him, whether or not I got better was far less important than the *profession* of the practitioner that got me better. Second, I realized that there were a lot of people—*highly educated people*—that had *opinions* about Chiropractic that were NOT formed from *scientific investigation.* Rather, these opinions were formed by *prejudice*; these opinions represented *dogma, not science.* Most tragically, these people were not afraid to offer their dogmatic, prejudiced opinions under the pretext that these were EXPERT opinions.

A few years ago, I received a phone call from the Washington State Chiropractic Association asking me to come down from Canada to lecture to medical students at the University of Washington School of Medicine. I had been the keynote speaker at their annual convention a few years earlier, and they felt that the scientific evidence I had gathered about the safety and effectiveness of Chiropractic was something that would be important to share with the medical students.

My experience had been that *evidence* was often the *last* thing used by most medical doctors to form an opinion about Chiropractic, and I just did not have any interest in participating. As a chiropractor, you sometimes just get exhausted from fighting prejudice all the time. I guess I was in a moment of fatigue.

I then got another phone call. This time, the caller was Dr. Gerry Clum, President of Life Chiropractic College West. (You will read his story in this book.) The Association had upped the ante! Dr. Clum personally asked me if I would participate. I told him what I had already told the people from the Association: I was simply not interested. BUT, I continued, if speaking at the Medical School was a personal favor to him, I would *consider* it. He replied, "Great, I'll have them call you to arrange your flight, and I'll see you there next week."

Before we speakers gave our lectures to the students, the medical doctor/professor who was the Head of "Complementary and Alternative Medicine" at the Medical School—and also the organizer of the event—briefed us. He started by saying that we should not worry about questions regarding *evidence* for what we do. He explained that the medical students were not aware that everything they did was not "proven." He told us that they would have a strong bias toward assuming that what they were learning in Medical School was *evidence-based* and that what all non-medical practitioners did *was not*. He said that we should just state that we were not there to prove anything or to provide evidence but, rather simply, to explain what we did and which patients we thought we could help.

I responded by saying that the *last* thing I was willing to do was evade a question regarding evidence or science because that would just perpetuate the dogmatic beliefs that most medical doctors held. I pointed out that, in fact, I had come to this medical school for the sole purpose of *correcting* that mistaken impression. I stated that this was *exactly* the right time to directly address such questions. In fact, I stated that I would NOT participate without the ability to discuss science and scientific evidence. The fact is: he ASSUMED that we did not have any scientific evidence. He ASSUMED that we would not be capable of answering these questions. He had the SAME belief system as the students, but disguised his prejudice with a condescending effort to protect us. Prejudice and dogma!

To make a long story short, we finally got into the classroom, and in came the group of medical students. I introduced myself, and said that I was there to answer any and all questions, that I was fully aware of some of the opinions that many hold about Chiropractic, and that I promised that they could not offend me by asking *any* question. In fact, they could only offend me by *not* asking a question. I said that *not* asking a question was offensive to me because it pre-supposed I could not answer it. Worse, it left the question unaddressed and denied me the opportunity to educate them. Furthermore, it denied them the opportunity to learn something they didn't know. I also stated emphatically that I was happy to learn from them and that any and all evidence that they had regarding any discussion was not only welcomed but encouraged.

The students looked at each other and sort of smiled as they prepared to pounce! Within a few seconds, the first hand went up. "We just came from anatomy class, and our anatomy professor told us how Chiropractic causes stroke; he showed us the vertebral artery and told us how Chiropractic adjustments can cause a tear in this artery. Is this true?"

I thanked the young student for her candid question. The first thing I asked was whether or not her professor had provided a single scientific reference supporting the conclusion that Chiropractic causes stroke. Of course, the answer was no. I then informed the students that according to the best research available—conducted by professors at the University of Calgary and published in the *Journal of Manipulative and Physiological Therapeutics*—that a Chiropractic adjustment does not even result in the loose tension being taken out of the artery, never mind any force being applied to it. A Chiropractic adjustment represents less stress on the artery than turning of the head in the normal range of motion.

I then told the students that I had published a commentary on the issue of Chiropractic and stroke in the same journal. In fact, *I gave them all a copy of it!* The article was a summary of all the available scientific evidence—as well as all the grossly negligent information that had been disseminated about Chiropractic and stroke. I told them of an article that was published in the *Canadian Medical Association Journal* that contained misleading information from a completely discredited study conducted by a Canadian neurologist who subsequently admitted—under oath—that he deliberately falsified data. This study formed the basis of a very organized and very negative anti-Chiropractic campaign in Canada. The entire campaign was based on misinformation—*deliberate* misinformation.

I also pointed out that the research clearly indicated that in the largest study ever conducted on the topic of Chiropractic and stroke, the authors found that less than 3% of strokes related to the vertebral artery even occur in people that have ever even seen a chiropractor and that no causal relationship between Chiropractic and stroke had EVER been established. Over 97% of all vertebral artery strokes occurred in people who had never seen a chiropractor, and nobody knew what caused these strokes—the vast majority were considered spontaneous!

I asked these students if it was scientific or logical to blame Chiropractic for any stroke when 97% of these strokes were caused by an unknown variable that was most certainly also present in the 3% of strokes that occurred in people who had seen a chiropractor. We all agreed that the scientific evidence pointed in the exact opposite direction of the prejudiced dogma that was both being published in the medical literature and obviously being taught at medical schools.

My presentation concluded after fielding several more questions, some about how Chiropractic works and some about which patients medical doctors should refer to a Chiropractor when they get in practice. I'm happy to report that the answers to these questions resulted in an even greater rapport with the students. I am encouraged to say that the students were very polite and respectful and that, after they realized that there was substantial scientific evidence regarding the safety and effectiveness of Chiropractic, they were also very willing to change their minds based on this evidence. At the end of the session, we all agreed that our moral obligation was to do the best for our patients, and that meant forming evidence-based opinions about all possible ways to help them.

My final words to the class were to have them promise that from that moment forward—every time they heard something negative OR positive about Chiropractic, or medicine for that matter—they would ask these most important questions: *"Where did you read that?"* and *"May I have a copy or the reference, please?"* I teach my patients to ask these questions; I teach chiropractors to ask these questions; given the rare opportunity to do so, I teach *medical students* to ask these questions; and I am urging you, the health- and wellness-seeking readers of this book, to ask these questions.

All I asked of those medical students—and all I ask of you—is to apply the same standard to all forms of healthcare. Don't allow dogma or prejudice to get in the way of promoting health or alleviating human suffering. Be a *scientist*, not a *cultist*.

Today, I tirelessly travel the world speaking at conferences and giving seminars for thousands in the hope that more and more people will avail themselves of the Chiropractic Wellness Paradigm. As you enjoy the stories in this wonderful book, *The Well-Adjusted Soul*, you will see for yourself the first-hand experience so typically enjoyed by those fortunate enough to have chosen Chiropractic as their health and wellness regimen. If you are currently benefitting from Chiropractic care, congratulations; if not, what are you waiting for?

James L. Chestnut, BEd, MSc, DC, CCWP

Chair—International Chiropractors Association (ICA) Council on Wellness Science

Developer and Lead Instructor— ICA Post-Graduate Wellness Certification Program

Board Member—ICA Committee on Chiropractic Postgraduate Education

President and Head of Research and Product Development— Innate Choice Wellness Nutrition

President and Head of Program Development— Eat Well Move Well Think Well™ Corp.

Developer of The Innate Lifestyle™ Program

Author of:

The 14 Foundational Premises of the Scientific Validation of Chiropractic

The Innate Diet®

Innate Physical Fitness®

The Innate State of Mind®

1

The Healing Power of Chiropractic

"The doctor of the future will give no medicine
but will interest the patient in the care of
the human frame, in diet, and in
the cause and prevention of disease."

Thomas Edison
Inventor
(1847-1931)

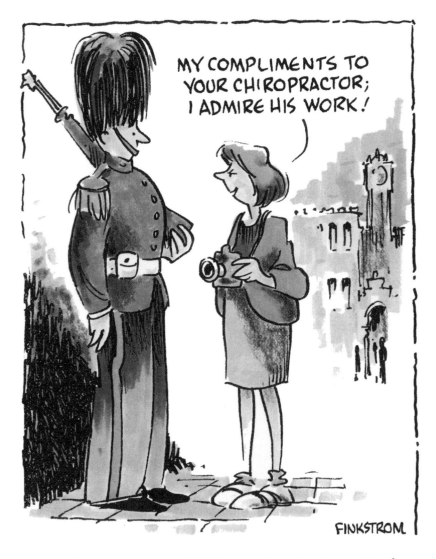

Reprinted by arrangement with Finkstrom Licensing International

Tack Room Adjustment

In the early 90s, I sold my Chiropractic office in La Jolla, California, and relocated not far from a small town in the Pacific Northwest. At the time, I planned on relaxing for a year or so on the horse ranch I had purchased before opening another practice. But as the beloved Scottish poet, Bobby Burns, put it more than two-hundred years ago, "...*The best laid plans of mice and men gang aft agley*...."

Operating a farm or ranch is physically demanding work, and country folks often sustain injuries from falling, lifting heavy objects like bales of hay, handling livestock, or myriad other causes. It wasn't long before my neighbors discovered that a chiropractor had moved in at the horse ranch. Soon, I found myself with a number of eager patients for whom I had made no plans. With the brisk, word-of-mouth patient-flow I experienced, I didn't even bother putting up a Chiropractic office sign at my driveway entrance.

The huge barn on my property housed stables for horses and a large tack room for storing saddles, stirrups, halters, bridles, and other gear. On an impromptu basis, I decided to allocate space in the tack room for adjusting patients. To the extent possible—on those days when I was seeing patients, I lined the walls with benches and chairs while I placed an adjusting table and a cervical chair in the center of the room.

In that rural environment, it was not unusual for patients I had already adjusted to hang around and watch me adjust their neighbors and friends before climbing back into their pickup trucks and heading home. After all, why watch "Reality TV" when you can watch "The Real Thing"?

Around seven o'clock one evening, I had already adjusted three patients and was about to treat my "last" one. (The previous three patients were still there.) I was interrupted when an unfamiliar voice hollered through the barn door near the parking area—about 30 yards from the tack room. A few minutes later, my patients and I saw a remarkable sight. Barefoot, and dressed in shorts and a tee shirt, a boy of about twelve had his left and right arms around the necks of his mother and father who were carrying him across the concrete floor. His legs were splayed, and each parent was holding one of his ankles. The weight of the boy's bottom was supported by his brother, about fifteen-years of age, waddling along, duck-like, "holding up the rear."

The first thing that struck me about the young man was that he was "way past his ego." Writhing in pain, his discomfort was so great that he had no energy with which to maintain an image or identity. His eyes were rolling back in his head. This was EXTREME kidney failure! My other patients in the tack room, as if in unison, issued a deep *gasp* when they saw the boy! Everybody was aghast at his condition and clearly concerned and uncomfortable with what they were witnessing.

In no time at all, my "last" patient pleaded with me to treat the young man right away: "Dr. Joe, take him...*please!*" I motioned for the parents to seat their child in the cervical chair. The boy's testicles were severely swollen and his legs were splayed to ease the pressure as he sat. Everything below his waist was throbbing. Under the fluorescent lights, his color was a bright, translucent yellow; he looked as though his skin had been sprayed with see-through yellow paint. Since he hadn't passed urine in days, his feet and legs were badly swollen—he looked like a Cabbage Patch Kid. The "whites" of his eyes were kind of a blood-tinged orange! I estimated he was carrying 20-30 pounds of excess fluid.

My one-and-only concern was, *"What is in the best interest of this patient?"* My first assessment of what I saw was, "This child needs to go to a *hospital...*NOW!" I had grave misgivings as to whether he could survive the night. Within moments, the boy's mother made it clear that she was the spokesperson for her offspring. I spent ten minutes trying to reason with her: "Your son's vital signs are rapidly deteriorating. He has severe edema. His kidneys have shut down and are backing up. He can't process any waste. His blood is badly poisoned. He needs to go to a hospital emergency room NOW or he will DIE before morning!"

The mother explained that the family had spent the previous four hours driving over winding roads through mountain passes in the Cascade Range from eastern to western Washington State—just to see *me!* She made clear that they were not opposed to medical treatment because of any religious beliefs. She told me they had heard about and seen enough instances of ineffective medical treatments at the hands of hospital doctors that they would only trust their son's life to a chiropractor. "Hospitals are where people go to DIE!" she stated in *don't-you-dare-argue-with-me* terms.

I can only conclude that the family had heard about my practice from one of my neighbors. What amazed me is that I was in a remote area in the middle of nowhere on a country road with no sign indicating that a chiropractor was located on the property! Somehow, they had found my driveway, my house, and then made their way to my barn—an incredible feat of night-time navigation! How could I *possibly* turn them away? The fact is: *I couldn't!*

I walked up to the boy and looked him straight in the eyes. It was one of those moments when you want to connect with a person soul-to-soul. I said, "Listen, I'm gonna' do my best to help you."

For some odd reason, at that moment there was a quiet debate going on in my head. Most of the time when a chiropractor considers intervention for the kidneys, he or she thinks, "T-12," the location of a critical vertebra in the *thoracic* part of the spine. But something told me this young man's problem was to be found in another part of his anatomy—his *cervical* spine, not far below his head! To this day, I don't know why that spot came to my mind. I then examined the patient with a Nervoscope, a hand-held electronic device that measures vertebral inflammation and gives thermographic (temperature) readings where there are subluxations (misalignments) in the spine. Lo and behold, he had a really HOT fifth cervical vertebra—"C-5" in chiropractor language. I then palpated the vertebra and determined that it was completely immobile. Obviously, *that* is the vertebra on which I performed my adjustment. Today, almost twenty years later, I can still remember that adjustment as the vertebra snapped into alignment—it felt like hitting a tennis ball in the "sweet" spot! It was one of those rare moments when *"you know that you know!"*

After my adjustment, I told the boy's parents to carefully monitor his kidney function and bring him back the next morning. They carried him past the stables, through the barn, and out to the parking area. As soon as they were beyond the door, the boy insisted that he be stood up in front of some bushes where he passed urine for the first time in five days. They spent the night at the home of a local friend.

When the family returned the next morning, I expected them to be carrying the boy into the tack room in much the same way he had entered the previous evening. Instead, I couldn't believe what I saw. The young man was a completely different person! He walked in under his own power. He was *normal!* His parents said that he had urinated about six times every hour throughout the night. It was as though the C-5 adjustment had reconnected the neurological circuit between his brain and his kidneys! He had absolutely no discoloration in his body. All his swelling was gone. The color was back in his face. His eyes were clear. It was as though he had never had kidney failure!

Ever since then, this boy—actually, he's now in his 30s—and his family, are still patients of mine. They still drive for four hours—each way—over winding mountain roads to get to my office, although I've since set up shop in a professional building in town and have a thriving practice. The "boy" is now a chef in a very nice hotel in Spokane. Every once in a while, in addition to visits for maintenance adjustments, I get letters from him letting me know how well he's doing and thanking me, basically, for saving his life.

That experience made a memorable impression on me. Since then, I've never underestimated the power of Chiropractic adjustment. Also, as a chiropractor, I believe in something we practitioners call "Innate Intelligence"—the power of the body to heal itself once nervous system interferences (subluxations) are removed. Even as a logical, intellectual, educated graduate of an accredited and highly-respected College of Chiropractic, I'm still amazed that a simple adjustment could have worked so fantastically well and so quickly. I was humbled by the speed and completeness of that young man's overnight recovery! To this day, with every single treatment, I strive to provide that same level of care to all of my patients, regardless of their condition.

Joe Dispenza, DC
Rainier Chiropractic Clinic
Yelm, Washington
As told to Don Dible

A Mother's Story

"My mother was the most beautiful woman I
ever saw. All I am I owe to my mother. I attribute
all my success in life to the moral, intellectual
and physical education I received from her."

George Washington
First President of the United States of America
(1732-1799)

One morning in the spring of 1927, a young, Munford, Alabama,
doctor offered this summary: "I'm sorry, but there's nothing else I
can do for her." Referring to their frail two-year-old, he told the
parents, "Just try and keep the child as comfortable as possible."

Without ceremony, the doctor placed his stethoscope back
in his black satchel and closed the clasp with a loud snap. To
the parents, it was as if the doctor had just pronounced a death
sentence on their little girl.

The child's father knelt by her bedside and broke into sobs.
The mother, tears streaming down her cheeks, continued to wipe
the child's body with a damp cloth.

"I'm *so* sorry," the doctor said as he turned and stepped
around the pail of soiled diapers. Pieces of sheets and assorted
cloths had been torn up for use as diapers. The diarrhea had
become severe; and the dehydrated child was so weak she didn't
have the strength to lift her tiny arms.

"There *has* to be someone—somewhere—that can help her;
there just *has* to be," the distraught father said as he lifted his
little daughter's limp body and cradled her in his arms. He
closed his eyes and cuddled her while he prayed: "Please, God,
we need Your help!"

A knock sounded at the front door. It was a neighbor that had gone out to his barn to check on a sick calf when he recognized the doctor's familiar horse and buggy passing by. The neighbor hurried over to find out what was wrong.

"Is everything okay?"

"Our daughter has diarrhea really bad, and we can't stop it. The doctor says there's nothing we can do for her."

"Yes, there is!" the neighbor said. "Dr. Joseph Barnett in Anniston is a chiropractor; and I'm certain that he can help. I'll get a horse hitched up to my buggy and come back straight away and take you."

"We're desperate; we'll try anything!" the father said. His swollen red eyes and the drained look on his face left no doubt as to the depth of his anguish. Both parents wasted no time in preparing for the nine-mile journey.

Hours later, traveling over rain-rutted dirt roads, the Good Samaritan neighbor delivered the child and her parents to the chiropractor's office. The look on the parents' faces told the doctor that this child had immediately become his priority patient!

Dr. Barnett examined—and then adjusted—her tiny body, explaining to the parents everything he was doing and why. Having had no prior experience with Chiropractic, the parents were astounded by the clarity and sensibleness of the doctor's explanations.

When the adjustments were completed, the father asked, "Will you need to see her again?"

"I don't think that will be necessary," the doctor replied as he handed the child to her mother. "She'll be fine now."

On the way home, the parents were shocked when their daughter opened her eyes, sat up, pointed out the buggy window, and smiled.

Dr. Barnett was right. The child's parents didn't have to take her back for another adjustment. She made a full recovery!

This story was told to me by my father—*I* was that two-year-old!

And how, you may ask, have I shown my gratitude to Chiropractic? I've given the world an *outstanding* chiropractor: my son, Dr. Gerald R. Kreitz!

Polly Camp Kreitz
Proud mother of
Gerald R. Kreitz, DC
San Antonio, Texas

Mrs. Kreitz is the author of
Magnolia Meadows, a novel

Release from an Emotional Prison

On an overcast afternoon, I walked into the reception room and saw my patient Nicole with one of her foster children, an old man in a twelve-year-old frame. His body was hung loosely, like a robe draped over the back of a chair. I approached the boy and, as I did so, he lifted his head but couldn't look me in the eye or stand completely upright. When I got closer, he reached out, grabbed my tie, pulled me in tight, and said, *"Hi, my name is Aaron."*

I was blown away. At that moment, I felt as if my only purpose in life was to help this boy. I asked Nicole for permission to examine him and, because she trusted me, she agreed. His story was disturbing. You can't imagine what I found during my case history and Chiropractic exam. You see, Aaron had spent the previous two years locked in a dark, damp closet. It was the way his birth parents chose to "teach him a lesson." He couldn't carry on a conversation and had severe learning challenges. His back was rigid and riddled with misalignments. He had adapted to two years of physical and emotional trauma by assuming a standing fetal position.

As chiropractors and Chiropractic patients, we are probably the only health care providers and consumers who truly understand that this was Aaron's innate way of protecting himself from the emotional pain of abandonment. Nicole told me that her previous chiropractor had said it would be a waste of money to treat the boy because he had no real symptoms.

Holding my rage inside, I said, *"I understand."* I lied! I asked Nicole if she'd like to hear *my* opinion. I told her what *you* would have told her, *"Aaron may not have the typical symptoms, but he has signs, and plenty of indicators, of what we call multiple subluxations. And there is a chance I might be able to ease his suffering; would you like me to try?"*

To Aaron and his foster family, the subsequent series of spinal adjustments were much more than mere treatments. I don't fully understand how, yet his foster parents and I witnessed firsthand the boy's release from an emotional prison. As a matter of fact, the adjustments kicked the door wide open! Six months later, Aaron was mainstreamed into school. No, he didn't rise to the top of his class; and yes, he still has challenges…but he no longer *suffers*.

No one healthcare profession has *all* the answers, yet what we do as chiropractors *matters* to our patients. There are hundreds of thousands of people that suffer needlessly every day and will continue a life of drudgery and hopelessness unless each and every chiropractor stands up and *shouts* the praises of our glorious profession!

Frank Sovinsky, DC
DC Mentors
Tahoe City, California

Dr. Sovinsky is the author of
Life the Manual:
When the pursuit of happiness makes you miserable

The Wiggles

Annually, more than one-and-a-quarter million children in the United States under the age of five require emergency room treatment due to falls.

Children's Hospital Boston

It was a quiet Wednesday afternoon last autumn when little Stacy entered our Chiropractic office cradled gently in her daddy's burly arms. Mommy completed the trio, carrying a large bag of toys, picture-books, and other stuff necessary to sustain a tot in the grip of something awful, but-as-yet-undiagnosed. The two-and-a-half-year-old, dressed in fresh, pink jammies with her long brown hair partially covering her face, was unconscious—limp as a rag doll.

The distraught parents explained that the previous Sunday they had discovered their only child writhing on the living room carpet—twisting and turning in uncontrollable spasms. Apparently, she had fallen off the couch. They wrapped Stacy in a protective blanket, set her in the cab of the family pickup, and rushed her to the emergency room. From there, she was promptly admitted to the hospital for observation.

A full complement of tests followed: blood pressure and pulse were checked, the pupils of her eyes and her ear canals were examined, blood was drawn and analyzed, x-rays were taken, and, ultimately—under sedation—a CAT-scan was performed. Try as they might, however, the hospital physicians were unable to identify the malady that was tormenting the child.

To stop the spasms—and to keep Stacy from injuring herself as she flailed her arms and legs, the best the doctors could do was administer high-powered pain killers—Valium and Phenobarbital—intravenously. In other words, the only physician-approved way little Stacy's spasms could be stopped was to put her into something very close to a coma—*continuously*. After three days of diagnostics, the doctors told the parents there was nothing more they could do. Armed with prescriptions for more pain killers—in oral form, this time—Stacy's parents were told to take the child home, put her to bed, and hope for the best.

Far from satisfied with this pharmaceutically-driven plan, Stacy's parents wisely decided to explore other options. After all, they had nothing to lose. Following the recommendation of friends, they chose our practice to see what, if anything, could be done to stop the spasms.

After discussing Stacy's condition with her parents for almost half an hour, I asked her father to place the child on her side on the adjusting table with her head and neck slightly elevated on the headrest. By this time, Stacy's pain killers had begun to wear off and she appeared to be quite groggy.

So that you may more clearly understand what happened next that fateful Wednesday afternoon, bear with me while I provide a short, technical explanation. Every chiropractor knows that muscles—and muscle spasms—are controlled by nerves that run through the spine. Therefore, I examined the entire length of Stacy's back—vertebra by vertebra—with my fingers (a process known as "palpation"). In no time at all, I discovered that the first vertebra in the upper spine—located just below the base of the skull and called "C-1" or the "Atlas" because it supports the globe of the head—was seriously out of alignment with the base of the occipital bone (skull), the opening through which our nerves leave the brain stem and enter the spine. This misalignment was responsible for pinching Stacy's nerves and causing her uncontrollable muscle spasms.

Having made that straightforward diagnosis, the next step was to execute a Chiropractic adjustment known today as a "hole in one," originally developed by B. J. Palmer, the acknowledged "Developer of Chiropractic." During my first adjustment attempt, I placed my left thumb at C-1 on the right side of Stacy's small neck, placed my right thumb on top of that, and applied pressure in an effort to move C-1 laterally into alignment with the base of the occipital bone. No luck. I next repeated the process while applying still more pressure. Again, no luck. Finally, on the third try, I heard a satisfying "squish" as the alignment of Stacy's spine was restored.

As soon as I completed the hole in one adjustment, Stacy instantly emerged from her stupor. She opened her brown eyes w-i-d-e, looked around at my unfamiliar office, and threw her arms in the air in the universally-recognized "pick me up" gesture. Daddy, who had stood by my side during the entire procedure, wasted no time in scooping up his little angel. Absolutely no sign of Stacy's previous spasms could be seen; she had recovered completely!

Moments later, her teary-eyed mommy retrieved a small security blanket from the tote bag and placed it in Stacy's hands. Mercifully, everything was back to normal.

Overwhelmed by the speed and full extent of their child's recovery, Stacy's choked-up parents did their best to explain to her how I had managed to stop "The Wiggles." Encouraged by her parents, Stacy decided that I was someone to be trusted—not feared. With a little more coaching from mommy and daddy, the still-shy Stacy was even persuaded to say, "Thank you, Dr. Cody!"

In my many years of practice, this is the closest I have ever come to seeing a miracle first-hand.

EPILOGUE

Since this extraordinary episode in our office, we have received several visits from Stacy and her father. It turns out that Stacy's daddy was so profoundly moved by the events on that special Wednesday he is now studying to become a chiropractor himself!

Cody J. Masek, DC
Complete Health Chiropractic
Temecula, California
As told to Don Dible

It Wasn't the Flu

Something bothered me when the receptionist at the office I worked in told me she couldn't have children. She and her husband had been trying for four years and seen many doctors including fertility specialists. They all said that while they didn't know what was wrong, the couple would never have children. I had just graduated from Chiropractic College and was the new doctor in the office. I couldn't believe that she had never had her spine checked for nerve interference. But she only believed in the effectiveness of Chiropractic for treating back pain...and she didn't have any back pain!

A few months later, her husband came by to pick her up from work one night, and I persuaded them to let me check their spines. I found nerve interference in her lower spine, the area where the nerves that supply her ovaries exit, and in her husband's first spinal nerve in the neck. I felt confident that these interferences were the reason why they couldn't have children. I didn't say that to them because they wouldn't have believed me, a new doctor who had just graduated from Chiropractic College. So, I just asked them to let me correct the nerve interference I found. "It only takes a minute," I said. "Plus, you'll be helping me to keep up my skills." They finally agreed, and three-nights-a-week, I brought them both into a treatment room and adjusted their spines.

Then one day, the receptionist called in sick. She said she had the flu. The next day, she called in again saying that she didn't know what was wrong with her. She had started feeling better yesterday afternoon but felt sick again this morning. I told her to buy a home pregnancy test and then told her why I thought she hadn't been able to get pregnant.

When she called back later that day, she was crying. "All the doctors told me that I would never have a family," she said.

"All but one," I replied. "I always knew that you would."
"It's a miracle," she cried.
"Yes, I know it is," I agreed, "a Chiropractic miracle!"
Nine months later, she gave birth to a very healthy eight-pound boy who, today, is five-years old.

Richard J. Parenti, DC
The Un-Chiropractor
Cary, North Carolina

2

Paths to Chiropractic

•

"Are you bored with life? Then throw yourself
into some work you believe in with all your heart,
live for it, die for it, and you will find happiness
that you had thought could never be yours."

Dale Carnegie
Author of *How to Win Friends and Influence People*
(1888-1955)

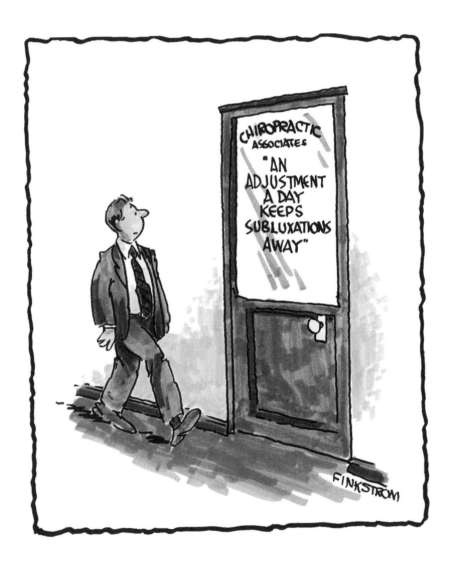

Reprinted by arrangement with Finkstrom Licensing International

Breath of Life

"Your first breath took ours away."

Anonymous

Given the opportunity to share a positive Chiropractic experience worthy of being published, I was flooded with memories of the past twenty years. In that time, I've had the privilege of personally touching the lives of more than twelve-thousand patients. Choosing just one story from thousands was a challenge. As you read my selection, you'll smile a knowing smile and understand why *this* is my hands-down favorite.

My life was changed forever when I was studying pre-med and running on the track team in college. One day I was sitting in my car at a stoplight when a drunk driver rear-ended me at high speed. I must have lost consciousness for a few moments, because I woke up staring at the ceiling of my car. Gathering my wits, I looked around to find I was in the middle of a busy intersection. I also noticed I was struggling to breathe.

Paramedics arrived at the scene, put me in a cervical collar, and whisked me away to a nearby emergency room. In the hospital, x-rays were taken and an exam was performed revealing that nothing was broken. Painkillers and muscle relaxants were prescribed, and I was told to go home. When I asked about my breathing difficulty, the doctor had no reply other than, "You're fine; just take the pills and you'll be good as new." Two weeks later, I was still suffering from severe neck pain and difficulty breathing. This made it impossible for me to compete in the 400-meter events…or even to train at all.

My father suggested that I visit a chiropractor. Ironically, he was raised getting regular Chiropractic care in the 1930s and

40s and would occasionally visit a chiropractor when I was growing up in the 60s and 70s. I say ironic because he never took any of his nine children to a chiropractor. I admit I was a bit skeptical about his suggestion.

When I actually *did* see a chiropractor, he described the connection between the spine and the lungs; he suggested that the accident might have caused misalignment in my neck; and he concluded that this was the probable cause of my difficulty breathing. His explanation was so logical that I agreed to let him "adjust" my spine. He then performed a quick and gentle adjustment to my neck. Much to my amazement—almost instantaneously—I was able to breathe fully again for the first time in two weeks. Not only did this enable me to again focus on my studies, I was also able to resume competition in track. The experience impressed me so much that I decided to change my academic program from medicine to Chiropractic. Fortunately, the pre-med coursework I had completed was the same as that required for the study of Chiropractic.

Upon graduation from the Parker College of Chiropractic in December 1992, I practiced in Connecticut for eighteen months before moving to Portugal. On September 17th, 1994, Chiropractic dramatically changed my life—once again. It was on that hot September day in Lisbon, Portugal, that my son, Christopher, was born. My wife and I were preparing and hoping for a home birth. Due to prolonged labor and the risk of medical complications caused by a previous C-section, our doctor suggested we go to the hospital for another C-section. My wife was emotionally devastated—for nine months, she had looked forward to a home birth and wanted no repetition of the complications of her first institutional delivery.

We rushed to the hospital for the procedure. Although I was asked to wait outside the operating room during the delivery, I was dressed in a surgical gown—ready to assist at a moment's notice. A short time later, my wife had a negative reaction to the anesthesia and her heart nearly stopped. Christopher was delivered, and one of the nurses urgently called me into the operating room. My wife was shivering uncontrollably, and the primary doctor said, "We almost lost her...." Not exactly words of encouragement and confidence.

The nurses were struggling to get Christopher to start breathing while the doctors attended my wife. The nurses had suctioned Christopher's mouth and spanked his behind but had the look of panic on their faces when they realized he wasn't crying *or* breathing. He looked blue, slimy, and limp; and his barely-open eyes were rolling in his head. Without hesitation, I took Christopher in my hands and did the only thing that came naturally to me. It was as if some mysterious force had taken possession of my body. I held my son's limp little body in my hands and cradled his tiny head with one hand. I adjusted his atlas—the first bone in the spine that supports the head. I used a technique I had learned personally from the late Dr. Larry L. Webster* just three years earlier. Once again, to my complete amazement, Chiropractic worked in a miraculous way. Christopher arched his little spine, stretched his arms and legs, and took a huge breath for the first time in his life.

It was on this day that I became a *real* Chiropractor. Before then, I had just *thought* I understood what it was to be a Chiropractor—treating a lot of people with low back pain, neck pain, those suffering injuries secondary to auto accidents, and other patients on a daily basis. On September 17th, 1994, I was powerfully reminded about *why* I had chosen to be a chiropractor. It was not pain, but rather the inability to breathe and perform, that originally led me to see a chiropractor. That changed my life completely. On *this* September day, the power of Chiropractic saved the life of my Christopher. The adjustment reconnected his nervous system to function better, as if by flipping a switch. As B. J. Palmer—the Developer of Chiropractic—observed: "The Power that made the body, heals the body, from above down, inside, out, and it doesn't happen any other way." Chiropractors save lives every day. My son is alive because of Chiropractic. If a Chiropractic adjustment can save a life, just imagine what it can do to keep you and your loved ones healthy.

Andrew P. Hatch, DC
CEO, Global Wellness
Sacavém
PORTUGAL

*Larry L. Webster, DC (1937-1997)

Dr. Larry Webster, the "Grandfather of Chiropractic Pediatrics," was a 1959 graduate of the Logan College of Chiropractic in Chesterfield, Missouri. In 1975, he founded the International Chiropractic Pediatric Association (ICPA), a non-profit organization dedicated to providing education, training, and support research on Chiropractic care in pregnancy and throughout childhood because "all children need Chiropractic care." Today, the ICPA serves more than 2,000 members worldwide. In addition to his work with the ICPA, Dr. Webster served the Life College of Chiropractic in Marietta, Georgia, as a pediatric instructor for eleven years, a clinic director for eleven years, and an associate professor. He also served on the post-graduate faculties of several Chiropractic Colleges including the Parker College of Chiropractic where—in 1991—Dr. Andrew Hatch was one of his students.

Another Chance at Life

"Ring around the rosie
A pocketful of posies
'Ashes, Ashes'
We all fall down!"

Nursery Rhyme
Anonymous

As a child, I always enjoyed being outdoors and sharing activities with my family. I remember one outing in particular that changed my life. I was six-years old, and my parents decided we should all go for a hike in the woods of Washington State. We came upon an old grist mill on a ledge by the Lewis River and decided to go down to the riverbank from there and play for a while.

There were two routes to get to the river. One was a well-worn trail behind the mill with thick limbs on each side, and the other—more adventurous—route involved climbing down boulders to get to the bottom. We decided to take the boulder route. My dad went down part of the way and positioned himself to help the rest of us. I—always the eager one—decided to go first. When I started, my foot slipped on some wet moss and I fell a full eighteen feet screaming, "Daddy! Daddy!" the whole way down. I landed on my head.

For a few minutes, I didn't move. My dad started to pray, "Jesus, don't take her." After the third prayer, I finally came to and cried. After an eternity, I started to move, and my dad climbed down to help me. My family then made a human rope to get me back up to the ledge. I remember my dad's white shirt was all bloody due to profuse bleeding from my forehead.

At the hospital, the gash on my head was stitched up. It wasn't until my mom begged the chief of staff to x-ray my arms and legs that it was discovered both my arms were broken. The doctor didn't bother x-raying my back, or running a CT-scan on my head. I was released shortly thereafter without any neurological examination.

Three months later, I started complaining of severe back pain. My mom would rub my back for hours to try and get the pain to subside. Nothing seemed to work.

About six months later, a lump appeared under my chin. My mom took me to five different medical doctors and their five separate opinions all resulted in the same diagnosis: I had a *thyroglossal duct cyst*. Five different medical doctors also recommended the same treatment: surgical removal. My mom was hesitant and decided to take me to a chiropractor, Dr. Randy Norris, for one last opinion. (If you're counting, that totaled *six* opinions!)

After taking x-rays of my back, the chiropractor found a total of *seven* abnormal curves, one of which was at the base of my spine. He started Chiropractic care immediately and my back pain began to decrease. After several months of therapy, my spine was once again straight, my pain was *history*, and the cyst under my chin disappeared and has never been seen since!

My mom told me a few years later what Dr. Norris had told her after first analyzing my spine. He said that I may have become severely crippled from the curves in my back if the problem hadn't been corrected before my teenage years. Furthermore, he said, without Chiropractic treatment, I probably would never have been able to bear children.

During my college undergraduate years, robust health permitted me to be active in a variety of sports including soccer. After graduation, I decided to enroll in Chiropractic College because I wanted to give someone else a new life with help from Chiropractic care the way Dr. Norris did for me. Today, I'm happily married to Dr. Scott R. Lenz, a fellow chiropractor. It is our privilege to care for the good folks in and around Eagle Point, Oregon. I thank God for my new life, overall well-being, and the opportunity to serve others—all due to Chiropractic.

Leigh Frisbee Lenz, DC, CVCP
Lenz Chiropractic
Eagle Point, Oregon

Crohn's Disease? Not Here!

Zabrina, one of my many nieces, got married about sixteen years ago. Since she is the daughter of an in-law, and given that ours is a fairly large family, I was not in attendance at her wedding. (Does that make her a "niece-in-law"? I'm not quite sure.) Nor was I immediately aware of the health problems she started to experience about a month after her nuptials. It was not until two months after the onset of symptoms that I became involved.

Soon after her wedding, Zabrina started to suffer severe stomach cramps and couldn't keep any food down. On the advice of a close member of her new husband's family, Zabrina was taken to see a medical doctor who was known to have helped several patients with stomach disorders. After multiple examinations and tests, the doctor diagnosed her with Crohn's disease. He prescribed a series of medications and placed her on a strict diet consisting of nothing but soup because, he said, she couldn't process normal food.

After a few weeks on the medications and the strict diet, Zabrina's condition did not improve; in fact, it got worse. Her husband took her back to see the family-recommended medical doctor who then reexamined her. He determined that her condition had escalated to "severe" Crohn's disease and would require hospitalization. In the hospital, she was subjected to extreme measures in the hope of curing her illness. What Zabrina and her husband thought would be a few days in the hospital turned into eight weeks at which point there was still no prospect of recovery.

The primary medical doctor placed her on several new medications, stopped feeding her—he said Zabrina couldn't process "real" food—and provided her with a saline-glucose IV drip which became her only source of nourishment. When no improvement resulted, he authorized examinations by additional doctors. A *series* of specialists, in turn, each prescribed more and more medications. One-by-one, each specialist assured the newlyweds, "This 'new' medicine will do the trick." The primary doctor even went to the outrageous extreme of requesting that a *psychiatrist* evaluate Zabrina because, he said, the problem was in her head! Now let's just think about that for one second.... If the problem was in her head, then why had she endured eight weeks of hell in the hospital under numerous medications? For Zabrina's husband, prescribing a psychiatric examination for his new bride was the last straw!

As word of Zabrina's declining health spread around my family and hers, I was made aware of her condition for the first time and promptly offered my services. My gesture was greeted with the usual "look-a-gift-horse-in-the-mouth" response. The newlyweds couldn't understand how a chiropractor—a "back doctor"—could help Zabrina. After all, the problem was in *her stomach*, not *her back!* On the other hand, the medical profession had totally dropped the ball, and the couple was ready to try anything to help the new bride of twelve weeks. (Remember, she had spent the last eight of those weeks in the hospital!) Zabrina's husband called me and accepted my offer of assistance. I wasted no time in presenting myself at the hospital.

Now this part is a scene right out of an action movie. Zabrina's husband stood by the door (keeping lookout) and watched for any hospital staff—"hostiles"—while I adjusted her spine. When I finished, I told her husband, "We need to get Zabrina out of this hospital, off the medications, on a program of Chiropractic care, and on a strict diet." But this time, the diet would consist of fresh vegetables, juices, and herbal teas. For a moment, Zabrina's husband thought his ears were deceiving him. I later explained that her stomach was in severe cramping because she hadn't had food in it for more than eight weeks. Her stomach was protesting this cruel and unusual punishment!

When Zabrina got out of the hospital, the couple thought her health issues were solved. However, the doctors had left her a small present: *drug withdrawal problems* that resulted in mood swings, hallucinations, loss of memory—for a short time she didn't recognize her husband, and more! However, after maintaining a steady Chiropractic program, a new, healthier diet plan, and lots of love, my niece recovered completely. To this day, sixteen years later, Zabrina has *never* had a symptom remotely resembling Crohn's disease!

Brian O. Burns, DC
Burns Family Chiropractic Center
Tampa, Florida

From Nun to Chiropractor

In New Haven, Connecticut, three-month-old Barbara suffered from a severe case of pneumonia. She was nursed back to health with love and care, only to be diagnosed with asthmatic bronchitis a short time later. Through the years, there were many sleepless nights—not just for Barbara, but for her parents, her four sisters, and her brother. In spite of visits to pediatricians, allergists, and emergency rooms—and in spite of experiments with medications, plastic breathing tents, and anything else that could possibly help Barbara's condition, no real progress was made.

After many tests, Barb's parents were told that she was allergic to dust, dog dander, mold, grasses, trees, and ragweed. Allergy shots were prescribed, and, once-a-week, Barbara would ride on the bus to the allergist's office for her dreaded shot. What a chore it was, just walking from the bus stop and up the stairs to the doctor's office. Barbara's wheezing and coughing could be heard by everyone as she entered the office. Week after week, month after month, her asthma continued. There were constant absences from school, excuses from gym classes, and class trips that could not be attended. Barbara loved baseball and wanted desperately to play with the neighborhood kids but, because of her asthma, had to sit on the sidelines and watch.

One day, after a severe asthmatic attack and a visit to the allergist, Barb's mom cried with fear, wondering what would become of her child. She questioned the allergist as to "what to do next." Surprisingly, the allergist told Barbara's mom to take her to a chiropractor, but made her promise never to tell anyone that he had recommended this. Elated over something "positive" for Barb's future, she immediately called Dr. Lewis Welch from a nearby town. No one in the family knew what a chiropractor was; but if there was any hope of relief for Barb, it didn't matter. Dr. Welsh arrived at Barb's home and asked that the cushions from the living room couch be arranged on the floor. He took out a black wax pencil and a little meter—called a Nervoscope—and had Barbara lie, face down, on the cushions. He ran the Nervoscope the length of her spine, watching a needle move from side to side and marking black spots on her skin. After this was done, he began his "Chiropractic adjustments" by moving individual spinal segments (vertebra) with his hands to restore nerve flow to various parts of the body. Barbara felt almost immediate results—a loosening in the chest and relief in her breathing. At ten-years of age, she felt that her life was just about to begin! After a series of "adjustments," Barbara began playing baseball with her sisters, brother, and friends. Gradually, gym classes were resumed. Autumn came and went—as did the pollen season, but there were no asthma attacks. It was almost too good to be true; so the hopes of Barbara's parents were not raised too soon for fear this relief would only be temporary.

Years went by, and Barbara entered high school. As her senior year approached and decisions for the future were to be made, Barb wanted very much to become a chiropractor, only to realize that the expense could not be met by her large family. Feeling a great need to serve in some way, and being active in the local Catholic Church, Barbara applied for the novitiate at Mt. St. Mary's in Newburgh, New York. For the next five years, she trained to become a sister of St. Dominic, took her vows, and began teaching school. Her missions included teaching in New Jersey and North Carolina. She taught first and fifth-to-ninth grades during her fifteen years in religious life.

During the summer of 1968, Barb spoke with Drs. Nelson and Helen Peet from Newburgh, New York, with whom she had become acquainted. She discussed her desire to become a chiropractor. The Peets, who were on the faculty at the Columbia Institute of Chiropractic in New York City, spoke to the president of the institute, Dr. Ernest Napolitano, about the possibility of Barbara's studying Chiropractic. Soon after, a presentation was made to her by Dr. Napolitano for a full, four-year scholarship. Life was about to change once more for Barbara, that little asthmatic from New Haven, Connecticut. She worked very hard to earn her Chiropractic degree so she could help others.

I am that little asthmatic from New Haven, and I have been in practice for 37 years. During that time, I have adjusted thousands of patients including infants, children, and adults who have responded well to Chiropractic care. What a wonderful feeling, to adjust the spine of an asthmatic child over a period of time and have them receive complete relief from these terrible asthmatic attacks. What a look of relief on the faces of their parents—the same look I saw that first day on the faces of my mother and father when Dr. Lewis Welch administered my first Chiropractic adjustment.

Barbara V. Thomas, DC
Thomas Chiropractic Office
Guilford, Connecticut

Path to Chiropractic

The four-year-old boy lived with his parents on the second floor of a north-side Chicago bungalow. Typical of the architecture, each of three, closely-spaced buildings bordered a common garden. The front door of the boy's apartment was reached by climbing a flight of steps to a small porch about six feet above the ground. At the time, the porch rail was badly rotted; and the landlord—in the process of repairing the rail—had removed the old one. The boy, unstoppably curious about the construction project, fell from the porch. How he missed the concrete sidewalk and hit a small spot of grass is still a mystery. Maybe little boys *do* have angels watching over them.

Although the boy survived the fall, he *did* land on his head! After hospital x-rays showed a hairline fracture of the skull, he was sent home as full of mischief as ever.

For a short time, the boy—whose mother called him Billy—seemed fine. Then the blackouts started. "No," the doctor assured the worried parents, "nothing is medically wrong." One day when Billy's mom found him passed out at the top of the steep flight of concrete apartment stairs, she became scared. She knew that—if Billy had blacked out—the fall could have caused serious injuries.

In seeking advice from a friend, Billy's mom was told about a local chiropractor. The friend advised that Chiropractic treatment was different and involved no drugs. She told Billy's mom about her severe headaches that had defied the doctors and had plagued her for years. The headaches responded—almost magically—to this new method. Billy's mom had exhausted all medical answers for his blackout problem when she arranged for an appointment.

The skilled fingers of the chiropractor soon located the tender knots beneath the skull on each side at the top of Billy's neck. The chiropractor explained that the fall had knocked the top bone out of place enough to press on the brain stem. He called this a spinal subluxation and, yes, this pressure on the spine was enough to cause the blackouts. After that first visit, the blackouts never came back.

By the seventh grade, Billy had missed a lot of school and—over the years—had a well-established pattern of health problems. He seemed to get every bug that went around. His asthma slowed him down a lot. The winters brought on one upper-respiratory infection after another. Penicillin, the newest wonder drug, was injected repeatedly with little effect—except that Billy developed a dislike for his doctor.

The doctor persuaded Billy's mom that her son—as well as his sister—would be considerably healthier without their tonsils. Since school was out for the summer, they both went under the knife on the same day. Billy's dislike for the doctor escalated to a much higher level!

Now without tonsils, Billy was sicker in the eighth grade than he had ever been and missed even more days of school! His infections, allergies, and asthma severely interfered with his life. His mother became disenchanted with the doctor, so Billy saw less and less of him and got fewer and fewer shots.

The next spring, Billy awoke for school one morning and discovered that his mother was unable to get out of bed. During the night, she had fallen on her way to the bathroom. Although she had made it back to bed, the pain in her lower spine would not permit her to sit, stand, or walk. It was then that Billy's mom remembered that the chiropractor from years earlier also treated back problems. Billy's dad called their old chiropractor and got a referral to one nearby. The new chiropractor made a house call that very morning. After examining Billy's mother, he was able to use his skill to relieve the pressure in her back, thus enabling her to once-again sit, stand, and walk.

Billy's dad had been in a bad car accident when Billy was in the seventh grade. Ever since, he had had terrible headaches from whiplash. The medical doctors had told Billy's father he would suffer headaches for the rest of his life and lose much of the mobility in his neck. Billy's dad began adjustments when he learned that whiplash responded well to Chiropractic treatment. Soon, Billy's dad was sleeping better, his headaches stopped, and his neck mobility returned to normal.

Naturally, after both his parents were helped by the chiropractor, Billy was taken to see him. After witnessing the miracles done for his mom and dad, and dimly remembering his previous chiropractor, he was quite willing to try this new doctor.

Billy's freshman year in high school was a milestone in many ways. He started seeing the chiropractor the summer before the start of classes and was under his care the entire year. While Billy's problems were not all cured by the following spring, a strange thing happened along the way. He didn't miss his usual thirty-or-more days of school. At the end of the year, he was awarded a certificate for perfect attendance—a lifetime first!

In the second semester of his freshman year, Billy's social studies teacher required him to write a paper on the career he wanted to enter. At that young age, Billy had no idea what he wanted to be; so his mom suggested he talk to the doctor about a career in Chiropractic. He gave Billy piles of books and literature that made writing the school paper a snap. Billy set his sights on what, at first, seemed like an impossible dream. He discovered that he would need two years of college-level liberal arts along with four-and-a-half years of Chiropractic College to earn his degree as a Doctor of Chiropractic.

One day—about a decade later, as Dr. Bill gently felt the tender knot at the top of the neck of a little girl that had been blacking out, he knew he could help. He knew what it could mean—not only in the life of the little girl—but also in the lives of the rest of her family. He also appreciated that all the effort of his previous ten years had been worthwhile.

If you haven't yet guessed, *I'm* Billy, and this is the story of my Path to Chiropractic. I've shared my personal experiences with you because you're special to me; and I want each of you to understand—as I do—the miraculous healing benefits offered by my proud profession!

William Charles Hollensed, DC
Dubuque, Iowa

A Handshake, a Hug, and a Very Special Adjustment

I am a chiropractor. It has been my good fortune to serve in this profession for almost forty years. Before that time, I was a Chiropractic *patient*—but not your *typical* patient, mind you!

My father suffered from occasional bouts of low-back pain. I remember when, as a child, being somewhat awestruck about a situation that could render this mountain of a man motionless and fearful to move. I also remember that, after he went to the chiropractor, he was fine; he was dad again.

About the time I was twelve-years old, I experienced a rapid, and rather severe, decline in my eyesight. As a kid, I didn't relate to my eyesight changing, but after several falls and a few broken bones, the orthopedist joked, "Maybe you should have the boy's eyes checked!" That's exactly what was done…and then things got *very* interesting.

From the first ophthalmologist, there was a second; from the second ophthalmologist, there was a neurologist; from the neurologist there was the Cleveland Clinic; and from the Cleveland Clinic there was a most disturbing diagnosis and prognosis. It seems that I was experiencing a condition known as "optic atrophy." The inside of the eye—where the nerve entered the eyeball from the brain—was showing signs of a considerable abnormality. The result was rather poor vision and an enlarged blind spot—a VERY enlarged blind spot. More importantly, the diagnostic "menu of maladies" included things like a possible brain tumor or multiple sclerosis. Obviously, these are things that no parent ever wants to hear about—and they especially don't want to hear that their child might have. My parents were frightened and didn't know what to do or who to turn to.

At about the same time, I went along with my dad for his regular visit to his chiropractor. We lived in Buffalo, New York, and the chiropractor practiced in Ontario, about thirty minutes from our home. The chiropractor, Dr. Cassan, was pleased to see my dad and asked him where he had been because it wasn't like him to miss his appointments. Dad related that we had been in New York City, and then in Cleveland, trying to learn more about what was going on with me.

My dad happened to be Dr. Cassan's last patient of the day; and after dad was adjusted, Dr. Cassan sat down with us and talked about what was going on with me. My dad was a smart man, but he was not a highly-educated man. No one had ever really explained what they thought was going on with me, what the words they were using meant, and what it could really mean for me in the long-run. That night, that is exactly what Dr. Cassan did! He explained what "bilateral optic atrophy" meant, explained what "idiopathic origin" meant, explained what "prognosis-unknown with a probability of further visual deterioration" meant. He then explained again to my dad— and, for the first time, to me—what he did as a chiropractor; and he suggested that we see if Chiropractic care might help me. I got my first Chiropractic adjustment that July evening!

Over the course of the summer, I saw Dr. Cassan two or three times a week. I watched the flow of people in and out of his office. I saw how much they appreciated his care and respected his opinion, and I saw how much he cared for them. As a young man, it was quite an education for me! After school started in the fall, we went back to the ophthalmologist.

After my pupils were dilated, the doctor zeroed in on my retina with his ophthalmoscope. As he was going through his examination, he suddenly asked my father "What have you done to this boy? This is a miracle!"

My father said, "We took him to a chiropractor."

The gentleman was not pleased and explained to my father in no uncertain terms what a mistake that was! His advice didn't go very far with his patient—or with his patient's father! He returned to his examination and found that the retina wasn't as pale as it had been before and my vision was much improved. In his mind, whatever had happened to me had NOTHING to do with the chiropractor. In my mind, what had happened to me had EVERYTHING to do with the chiropractor. Seated in that examination chair, in that ophthalmologist's office, there was one thing that I could see with crystal clarity: I would become a chiropractor!

I continued to receive Chiropractic care on a regular basis after that first summer, and my eyesight continued to improve over time. I didn't qualify for a driver's license until I was in my twenties—and there are some members of my family that don't think I qualify to this day!

Dr. Cassan became my mentor. As I got to know him better, I realized what a wonderful man he was. He was one of those professorial, grandfatherly, counselor-friend types that everyone who meets is attracted to.

Over the years, I came to appreciate what a powerful role Dr. Cassan had played in my life. As a sign of respect for the two most important men in my adolescence and young adulthood, I named my son Donald Cameron—Donald after my father and Cameron after my chiropractor. But it didn't stop there.

When my son, now a chiropractor-married-to-a-chiropractor, was a young boy, he also met Dr. Cassan and had the opportunity to know him differently than I did but in an equally special way. Since my father died when my son was very young, Dr.

Cassan became a surrogate grandfather, Pop-Pop Cam. When his first son, my grandson, was born, the boy was named Cameron Gerard—Cameron after Dr. Cassan and Gerard after me. At first, my son wanted to name him Gerard Cameron, but after some considerable amount of pleading, I convinced him Gerard was a tough moniker to grow up with and that Cameron was a better first name!

As an adult, I have thought back to those fateful days in that office in Ontario, and I have been so grateful for all that Chiropractic has given me—the changes in my eyesight and the introduction to a career were just the beginning. In the fullness of time, I have come to appreciate another great gift Dr. Cassan and Chiropractic care gave me.

On that summer evening many years ago when it was just the three of us in Dr. Cassan's office, I remember watching my father's face as the words, the concepts, and the possibilities about my health and circumstances were translated into terms my father could comprehend and appreciate. I now understand the change that came over my father's face that evening; it was the draining away of fear and anxiety about the wellbeing of his son that he had felt up until that moment.

My father and Dr. Cassan have both passed away, and my hair has turned gray. Two things I long for to this day would be one more handshake and a hug from my father and one more of those very special adjustments from my first chiropractor.

Gerard W. Clum, DC
President
Life Chiropractic College West
Hayward, California

3

Proud to Serve the Profession

"Pride is a personal commitment.
It is an attitude which separates
excellence from mediocrity."

William Blake
English poet, painter, and printmaker
(1757-1827)

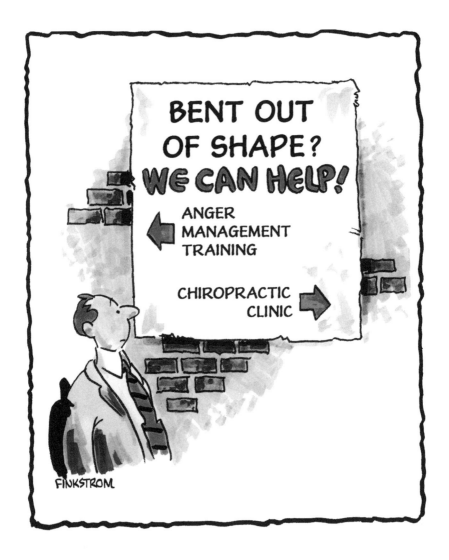

Reprinted by arrangement with Finkstrom Licensing International

The Day I'll Never Forget

I opened my Chiropractic practice in 1963 at the very young age of 21. It was eleven years after that—while attending a Chiropractic meeting in Atlanta, Georgia—that I experienced a life-changing paradigm shift. But before I tell you about my "shift," you need to understand my state of mind on that Day-I'll-Never-Forget in Atlanta.

I had been in practice for eleven years, and—truth be told—I was getting bored. While I was very thankful to have a successful practice, I found that the day-in-and-day-out merry-go-round of people, health complaints, and solutions was becoming all too common and routine. I asked myself, "Why am I traveling again from New York to Georgia to listen to other Doctors of Chiropractic talk about the need to serve more people? Why would I want more of the same?"

I sat in the back of the hotel ballroom filled with nearly 1,000 doctors, wives, husbands, students, and office staff. It was at a point in the program where specific doctors were asked to give short talks and tell how they were doing or share a particular case history. I half-listened while half-reading the program to see what was coming next. A young chiropractor from Canada, "Dr. Bruce," took the microphone and began to tell us of a new patient he had acquired since the previous meeting, three months earlier.

A 28-year-old, single, male parent, Jim, entered Dr. Bruce's office with a very painful, low-back complaint. Accompanying him was his seven-year-old daughter. The first visit consisted of an examination and evaluation. The young girl sat quietly and respectfully while her father and the doctor completed their time together. As Dr. Bruce said goodbye, the girl remained quiet and didn't make eye contact with him.

The next visit, Jim returned for the Report of Findings and to discuss his plan for Chiropractic care. Again, his daughter was with him. Again, she sat in the corner, saying nothing as Jim and Dr. Bruce discussed the results of the previous visit. Jim started care and received his first adjustment while his daughter watched.

As is normal, Jim saw Dr. Bruce three-to-five times in each of his first several weeks of care. And each time, he was accompanied by his daughter who sat and watched without saying a word. It was a Wednesday of week three, Dr. Bruce told the audience, when Jim laid down on the table and received his adjustment while his daughter watched. As Dr. Bruce raised the adjusting table for Jim to leave, the girl suddenly asked if she could be adjusted. Dr. Bruce was shocked. He asked her name.

"Jenny," she replied.

"Well, Jenny, you sure *can* be checked and adjusted—if it's okay with your dad."

Jim gave a shrug of his shoulders and an approving nod of his head.

Jenny approached the adjusting table.

"Jenny, I have to ask you a question," said Dr. Bruce. "Why, after all this time, did you decide you want to be adjusted? Do you have a back problem or pain?"

"No," replied Jenny. "I just wanted to because it must be good for you."

"How do you know that?" asked Dr. Bruce.

Jenny's reply shocked every single person in that Atlanta hotel ballroom: "Because, since my dad has been getting adjusted, he's stopped beating me."

Everybody in the stunned audience all realized—some for the first time—the full scope and effect of their mission to serve people through Chiropractic. That child's statement hit me hard. For more than thirty years of active practice after that, nothing was ever routine or "boring" again.

William C. Remling, DC (Retired)
Surprise, Arizona

The Proudest Day of My Life

My parents wanted me to be a "real" doctor. By that, they meant a person who prescribes drugs or performs surgery. While those measures are sometimes necessary to avoid impending doom, I knew there was something missing within that paradigm: Health and Healing. I researched Chiropractic, talked to people about Chiropractic, and discovered a real-life chiropractor in my neighborhood. He lived close by, and I'd occasionally pass him on the street. I was fascinated with him because he always seemed so full of life. You could tell; he loved what he did. I wish I could have said the same for almost everyone else I knew at the time.

After becoming Dr. Mark's patient at the age of thirteen, I was in awe of how I felt after my adjustments. After my first adjustment, I realized I was on a different path. My parents were supportive at first; but others I knew could not hold back their ridicule. My family doctor smirked and rolled his eyes at me when I told him of my interest in Chiropractic. Dr. Smith, a highly-regarded pediatric ophthalmologist at the Toronto Sick Children's Hospital, came to address our Baha'i community to talk about Spirituality and Faith in everyday life. When I took him aside to ask his opinion of Chiropractic, (For some reason, I thought he would be an expert.) he warned me of its dangers and how he had heard of countless devastating cases involving Chiropractic patients.

I was confused. Why the controversy?

Undaunted, and in the face of ridicule from both my family and my friends, I pursued an education in Chiropractic. As I did so, I could always sense a bit of resistance coming from my parents. During my year of graduation from Chiropractic College, I received a simple, devastating email from them: "Nima, when you are finished with your Chiropractic studies, if you want to go to medical school, you have our full support."

After eight years of Chiropractic study, they wanted me to do another eight years because what I had wasn't good enough????

That message lit a huge fire under my derrière.

Following graduation, I eventually moved to Maple Ridge in beautiful British Columbia, where I worked night and day building my practice and becoming successful. I desperately needed to show my parents that I could make it. I prayed for the day they would see that I was right in my decision. I'm forever grateful for their well-intentioned-but-negative push—the one that drove me to where I am now.

Well, that day finally did come. My parents were in town and came to visit me in the office. It was a busy Saturday afternoon, and they sat there in the reception room watching all these people come and go, patient after patient. I secretly was glad they stopped in on a busy day so they could see that, after all, I wasn't a disappointment to them.

I had finished seeing my last scheduled patient when a lady was literally dragged in—held up by her husband on one side, and a cane on the other. She was hunched over and asked if I would take in a new patient at the end of the day. How could I refuse someone who was obviously suffering so badly? I asked my parents to wait a bit longer while I looked after her. I swung her arm around my neck and shoulder and supported her while I dragged her into the consultation room.

I discovered that Gwen had been dealing with her affliction for two full weeks and hadn't slept at all in that time. However, her problems went much deeper. She had experienced excruciating back and sciatic pain for *years*, and her medical doctors kept prescribing anti-inflammatory medications, muscle relaxants, creams, and potions. She was even sent to an orthopedic surgeon who felt it was time to operate. Gwen was scheduled for surgery in six months, but her condition had worsened so much that she couldn't tolerate the pain and discomfort anymore. Against her doctor's recommendations (They told her *never* go see a chiropractor.), she ended up in my office at that exact moment.

My examination revealed that her L-5/S-1 and S-I (sacroiliac) joints were so locked up that it was clear they hadn't moved for years. Her x-rays showed severe spinal degeneration as well. This was a woman who clearly hadn't exercised, hadn't eaten appropriately (she was diabetic), smoked, and never took care of her spine or herself. She admitted that she had lived a difficult life, which told me that she was still holding on to psychological resentments from her past. Her joints through her neck and upper back were stiff and locked up as well.

I went right in there and put all my *focus* and *energy* and *intention* on bringing about order in all this "spinal chaos." When I adjusted her neck, her reaction was an instantaneous: "Oh my God, the room seems brighter!" She asked me why that would be, and the best explanation I could give was that her nervous system interference was preventing her body from working normally. My adjustments were permitting her nerves to reconnect, and those nerves were starting to function properly.

When I got to her lumbar spine, I put all my focus and intention on seeing a greater possibility of function. When my treatment was complete, Gwen got up off the adjusting table, stood up without any support of a cane or myself, and broke down in tears. In my office, this whole process of x-rays, examination, and adjustment took about half an hour.

Gwen then walked up to the front desk, without a cane, and continued to shed tears of wonder. She hugged her husband, who was crying as well.

It was that moment when I turned, looked, and saw both my parents in tears as they observed the whole thing.

In the coming weeks, I continued to work with Gwen to help restore proper function that had been out of balance for decades. In only six weeks of care, she was walking—full time—without a cane, something she hadn't done consistently in many years. Her doctors cancelled her surgery, and her husband also started care in my office, as did their daughter.

One day, when Gwen didn't show up for an appointment, we called to see where she was—and were saddened to learn that she had died of a heart attack. Her lifestyle choices had finally caught up with her. That was an "Aha!" moment for me, because it was then that I decided to start shifting my Chiropractic practice into more of a teaching facility—a setting where people would come to learn how to live healthier lives in mind and body, rather than simply try to "get rid of a pain."

Gwen was my greatest teacher, and the reason behind the proudest day of my life. I wouldn't trade that feeling for becoming a "real" doctor for all the money in the world.

Nima Rahmany, DC
Westgate Wellness Centre
Maple Ridge, British Columbia
CANADA

Touching Hearts and Minds

I didn't know anything about prenatal Chiropractic care twelve years ago when I was pregnant with my daughter. I also didn't know that a car accident eight years before she was conceived could affect her delivery. When I checked into the hospital three weeks before my due date to have labor induced, I expected my delivery to be perfectly normal and that everything would be fine. I was wrong.

Twenty seven hours after labor was induced, when four hours of pushing labor was having no results, my midwife went and got an obstetrician to consult on my case. He determined that Mikaela was stuck in the birth canal. My pushing wasn't moving her any closer to delivery, and her heart rate was decelerating to a dangerous level. The obstetrician asked us if he could use the vacuum extractor, although it wasn't really an option; he said they were losing Mikaela.

The doctors attached the suction cap to my baby's head and began pulling as I pushed. When her head cleared, I remember a short-lived sense of relief until the doctor informed us that Mikaela was wedged tight. Apparently, one of my hips hadn't spread properly—undoubtedly due to the earlier car accident, and there wasn't enough room for my baby's shoulders to get through.

The doctor informed my husband and me that he was doing everything he could, but that he was losing both of us. Then he reached in and wrenched Mikaela out. The rest is just a blurry nightmare. I went toxic at the moment of delivery, and Mikaela looked dead. I watched from across the room as two hospital personnel each held one of my baby's ankles and flicked the bottom of her feet trying to get her to cry. Mikaela never made a sound, and they rushed her from the room without bothering to tell me where they were taking her.

I refused treatment for the toxemia until someone told me what was going on with my baby. I remember lying in shock as a pediatrician that I didn't know gave me a sterile list of the problems facing my newborn. Her Apgars were 4 and 6; she was fighting for her life; she was on IVs and oxygen; and her left arm was completely numb. I asked the doctor if her arm was going to atrophy. He informed me that that was *the least* of Mikaela's problems; but, yes, it could. He said something along the lines of, "*If* she makes it, she'll need a couple of surgeries, and then she *may* regain *some* feeling in her arm."

This doctor was not Mikaela's pediatrician; Dr. Judi Krogstad was on vacation the night Mikaela was born, and this was one of her colleagues. I had researched pediatricians, and Dr. Krogstad was the best in the county; this guy, not so much.

We spent the next six days in the hospital recovering; and, upon her return, Dr. Krogstad saw Mikaela every day. My baby was slowly improving, but we still had several frightening moments. The first time Mikaela was brought to me, she was three days old; and two hours later, her body temperature had dropped to a dangerous level. I didn't even get to keep her with me until she was five days old. We were also having breastfeeding issues, but Dr. Krogstad was certain we just needed to get home and everything would work itself out.

The day we were released, Dr. Krogstad informed me that Mikaela was still in some danger and that she wanted to see her every day at 2:00pm for the next week—including Sunday.

The next day, I took Mikaela to her standing appointment; and Dr. Krogstad was pleased to hear that she had started breastfeeding as soon as we were home. The doctor was still concerned about the baby's color and ordered another bilirubin test. While this was being done, she informed me that Mikaela had a brachial plexus injury—damage to the network of nerves that sends signals from the spine to the shoulder, arm and hand. She wanted me to make an appointment for Mikaela to be seen by Dr. Claudia Anrig. I figured she was a pediatric orthopedist or neurologist; and Dr. Krogstad said, "No, she's a chiropractor." Well, I'm sure that I looked at her like she had just sprouted a second head out of her neck. That was *insane!* I told her I'd have to talk to my husband about it; but inside I was sure he'd think the concept was as crazy as I did.

My only experience with Chiropractic had been after my aforementioned auto accident. That man was not a very good chiropractor, so I had pretty much written off the whole profession.

When we got home that day and my husband called to see how Mikaela's appointment went, I told Michael about Dr. Krogstad's referral. He said to see if she was a provider on our insurance, like he was actually entertaining the idea. I was appalled.

The next day, Dr. Krogstad asked if I had called "Dr. Claudia" yet. I stalled. I told her I had to see if she was a provider on our insurance. She was.

The next day—and in the days following—I continued to stall. On the seventh day, when Mikaela was just thirteen days old, I took her to her final appointment. Dr. Krogstad took one look at Mikaela and said, *"This baby has not seen Dr. Claudia!"* I remember looking down, feeling a little ashamed of myself but also concerned that I had run out of excuses. When I looked back up, Dr. Krogstad was staring at me with steel in her eyes and said, "I have given you *sound medical advice*, and you're not taking it. Either you call Dr. Claudia Anrig *today* to make an appointment for this baby, or I'm going to report you." She was loud and vehement; and I stood there in shock.

Dr. Krogstad stomped out of the room; I dressed Mikaela and left. I cried all the way home, warring with my own fears. We got home, and I was still crying when my husband called at his usual time to check on the baby. He asked what was wrong with her, and I told him, "Nothing." So he asked why I was crying, and I told him, "Dr. Krogstad *threatened* me!"

I remember him asking why we had picked Dr. Krogstad. I told him she was the best pediatrician in the county. He said, "Well, if the best pediatrician in the county is this adamant about it, what's the problem?" Isn't it just like a man, to cut through all the emotional nonsense and get to the root of the matter?

So, I hung up and called Dr. Claudia's office. Over the next seven months, she helped us through constipation, ear infections, colic, and a horrible bout with thrush. Then one day, Mikaela raised both arms over her head for the first time. I cried! In that emotion-filled moment, I had *no idea* that this symbolic gesture would take on a life of its own, touching hearts and minds well into my baby girl's future.

It was just a few short months later that I made the mistake a lot of mothers make—I dropped out of Chiropractic care. Mikaela was all better—right? *Wrong!*

By the time Mikaela was three, she was suffering from allergies so bad she'd wake up gagging and vomiting from post-nasal drip. Mikaela was four when she started seeing Dr. Claudia again. Within a few years, no more allergies, no more annual colds, no more chronic ear infections...no more problems. Period!

But that's not where the story ends. I now work for Dr. Claudia, helping her help other Family Wellness Chiropractors have the same kind of relationship with their local pediatricians that she had with Dr. Krogstad. Through her mentoring program, I help her help other chiropractors educate their patients on the benefits of Chiropractic care for children. I travel around the country with her; and when I come home, the first question my daughter asks at the airport is *not*, "What did you bring me?" It's: "How many times did you tell my story, Mom?"

Mikaela knows how important her story is; she understands that more parents need to know this truth. The simple fact is: my ignorance could have cost my daughter the use of her left arm. Today—everywhere that Dr. Claudia and I are privileged to speak—Mikaela's story is touching hearts and minds.

Anastasia Line
Parent and Chiropractic advocate
Business Administrator
Dr. Claudia Anrig's
Family Wellness Resource Center
Clovis, California

My Solemn Promise:
I Will Try!

Around 6:30pm, as I arrived home after a busy day at the office, the ringing of my cell phone interrupted my stride.

"Hi, my name is Jill, and my mom and dad are patients of yours." Hearing despair in her voice, I recognized urgent concern. Being new in practice, I was eager to make a positive impact in peoples' lives; the opportunity presented itself that evening.

"My parents brought home a brochure from your office about infertility," Jill said. She went on to explain that after more than a year of trying, she and her husband were deeply concerned by her inability to become pregnant. She shared with me her discouraging experience of many evaluations and tests at a well-known fertility clinic. Her gynecologist had prescribed Clomid, a medication commonly used to stimulate ovulation.

Nothing was working. Their hope of becoming parents diminished daily. Infertility tugged at their hearts, causing not only emotional stress, but needless arguments within their otherwise-loving relationship. Jill was frustrated because she had been pregnant in a previous marriage, but conception was now eluding her and her new husband.

Jill concluded her call by skeptically asking, "Do you *really* think Chiropractic could *possibly* help me?"

I wanted to offer this young lady a solution, and the words of the late Dr. Fred Barge—a world-renowned Chiropractic author, leader, and personal mentor to me—echoed in my mind: *"You cannot promise* anyone *that you can cure them, but you* can *promise that you will* try!"

I responded frankly, "Jill, I can't guarantee that you'll become pregnant. In fact, Chiropractic doesn't *cure* anything. However, I *do* know this: the nervous system is the master control system of the body, and your body—everyone's body—is always striving towards health. If your problem is due to a vertebral subluxation—causing interference within your nervous system—that alone may be blocking your life-potential and inhibiting proper bodily function. By being adjusted, the interference will be removed, and there is a great chance your body will respond with restored function." My own words flooded my mind because, as I spoke, I had a tiny doubt as to whether Chiropractic would help her situation.

The next morning, Jill came to my office, and I led her through an entire new patient consultation. Feeling as though all of her hopes and dreams were placed on *my* shoulders, I explained Chiropractic, all the parts composing the nervous system, and how the nervous system helps to express LIFE!

I then asked, "Are you ready for your first adjustment?"

Jill nodded enthusiastically; in her desperation, she was willing to do *anything*.

In the still moment just before I delivered her adjustment, I let go of doubt. I focused inwardly and—with faith, connected deeply with my Chiropractic soul. I allowed Jill's Innate Intelligence to lead the way.

The anticipation for Jill to become pregnant built as she continued Chiropractic care with regular weekly visits. In just under two months, she arrived one afternoon bubbling over with vitality. Through tears of gratitude, she shouted: *"Dr. Eric, I'm pregnant!"*

As a chiropractor, even I had harbored uncertainty about the outcome of Jill's treatment. Her result is a testament to the power of the body and a salutation to the opportunity Chiropractic offers for living life to the fullest. I'm sincerely grateful for the lesson I learned, always remembering to carry *certainty* in my Chiropractic practice. Rather than a last resort, Chiropractic is the *primary option* for correcting and maintaining optimal health.

Eric Russell, DC
Beacon Chiropractic
Commerce, Texas

Associate Professor
Parker College of Chiropractic
Dallas, Texas

The Autistic Bicyclist

"As a full-time professional research scientist for 50 years, and as a researcher in the field of autism for 45 years, I have been shocked and chagrined by the medical establishment's ongoing efforts to trivialize the solid and compelling evidence that faulty vaccination policies are the root cause of the epidemic. There are many consistent lines of evidence implicating vaccines, and no even marginally plausible alternative hypotheses."

Bernard Rimland, PhD, Director
Autism Research Institute

It was a chilly fall afternoon when a local MD suggested that eleven-year-old Johnny pay a visit to our office. Johnny's mother cared so much about her little boy that she heeded the doctor's advice even though Chiropractic seemed p-r-e-t-t-y unconventional to her. You see, Johnny wanted to ride a bike awful bad since most kids his age were already doing it. But Johnny had a problem, and it wasn't with his back or his spine—he was *autistic!*

Autistic children have lots of trouble interacting with others—verbally, physically, *and* socially. The MD said that he had heard only good things about Chiropractic, and he told Johnny's parents they had nothing to lose. Though Johnny was sweet, he was a bit distrusting of our staff and doctor...at first. On the other hand, his mom was totally committed to seeing him succeed, so she agreed to the recommended treatment plan.

With more than a little trepidation, we began working with the boy. Johnny's spine was adjusted multiple times per week—daily, at the start of his Chiropractic care. We also did active therapy with him. The first active care session was interesting. We had a very large ball—about the size of a beach ball—and tried handing it to him. His poor coordination prevented him from holding on to it. But our Chiropractic Assistant was so patient that she and Johnny quickly developed a solid bond.

Each time Johnny came in, he was adjusted and then worked with the ball. It was frustrating at first since he was unable to hold it. Then Johnny had a breakthrough! One day, he grabbed the ball and held on for dear life! We also introduced a thick, red elastic band into his treatment. We wanted him to stretch it. Imagine the delight of our staff when, by the third week, he was exercising with the elastic band and pulling it all by himself!

We also stretched Johnny's muscles; and the results were amazing. We then started rolling the ball to him along the floor. It wasn't long before he could actually *catch* the ball. After more adjustments and more games of toss-the-ball, his nervous system began to function as it should and his coordination kicked in. That's when his healing *really* took off!

Johnny's mother said that even his *attitude* was noticeably different—she was *soooooo* encouraged. We went from tossing the ball to working on the coordination of his feet. We placed him on a stationary bike and helped him pedal by moving his legs for him. Naturally, this took a lot of time—and *even more* patience! Johnny's obvious excitement, however, made the patience easy. Clearly, he was making slow-but-sure progress.

Johnny's enthusiasm lit up our whole active care area; and patients just loved to come by and see how he was doing. Beaming with smiles, he'd clap his hands gleefully after every successful effort. By the end of each visit, it would be obvious that he was proud and happy...and verrrrrrrrrrry tired!

At this point, Johnny was well on his way to the hoped-for outcome. But he wasn't yet able to pedal the stationary bike by himself—until that special day. You can only imagine the emotional thrill of everyone in our office when he first pedaled without assistance. There wasn't a dry eye in our whole office. *Our little patient could actually ride a bike!* Suddenly, a life that neither he nor his parents dared ever dream of became a reality! You see Chiropractic is like that—the possibilities are endless when you just give the body the ability to work along with God's will to heal.

Lisa Speaks
Clinic Director of Projects and Strategic Planning
Parker College of Chiropractic
Dallas, Texas
and
Kirtland J. Speaks, DC
Expressions Chiropractic & Rehab
Cedar Hill, Texas

Sacred Mission

I was blessed with the opportunity to serve an extremely poor community in Fortaleza, Brazil, for a week. Many of my patients asked me what it was like, and I've had few words that could come close to describing the incredibly sacred, life-changing experience that it was for me.

Forty-two chiropractors, all of whom practice Chiropractic for the purpose of assisting people to become whole—physically, emotionally, mentally, and spiritually—by clearing the "static" in the communication within the nervous system, all traveled to Brazil together. We met in Miami and flew to Sao Paulo, Brazil, and then north to Fortaleza.

In Fortaleza, we slept and ate at a convent in the city; and each morning, we were transported to our adjusting destinations.

I arrived in the "ghetto" and applied my Chiropractic skills in a church. An extremely large, makeshift adjusting room over-looked the ocean. Each morning, the church was filled with more than 100 people. Some waited as much as two hours to be adjusted. These people were invited to return every day, some-times two times a day, throughout the week. The elderly, the women, the men, the teenagers, the young children, and of course, the babies, all filled the church. After school let out, children in uniforms lined the chairs waiting to be adjusted.

The tension in these people's spines was tremendous, and some had so much heel, ankle, and leg tension—indicative of spinal cord tension, that I could hardly move them. But, as the week progressed, profound changes occurred. An elderly woman told me that prior to starting her care, she had been unable to do anything in her home. After her adjustments, she was able to do *everything*. A little boy had recently fallen, he wore a bandage on his forehead, and his eye was swollen shut. Within two days, his eye was completely open and he was smiling again. On our last day, a man who had been in an accident twelve days earlier was carried in to our makeshift office in tears. He was adjusted each hour of the morning, and after the first adjustment, he could stand by himself. By the second hour, he could walk slowly, and by the third hour, he was laughing, smiling, walking, sitting, and his life was good again!

The changes and healing in many seemed remarkably fast. The energy in the huge adjusting room was powerful, peaceful, and full of God's presence. By the last day, we had received countless blessings, prayers, and thanks—in Portuguese, plus lots of hugs and kisses. We were grateful for our interpreters.

The community members came together on our last evening to celebrate their transformations—and ours. They wrote songs, danced with us, exchanged addresses, and took a myriad of pictures.

Leaving Fortaleza was difficult for us, and the community we established with these people felt like family. There was much love, no judgments, and plenty of giving and receiving by all. We shared a part of our souls with one another. Several of the chiropractors set up sponsorships for some of the children and their families for food, clothes, and school supplies. As you read this, I hope you are able to feel or sense the impact this has had on me. My wish for each of you is that you are able to experience the presence of God and your innate connection to humanity at the magnitude that I have been so blessed to receive in Fortaleza. Life will never be the same.

Lori L. Krauss, DC
Chiropractic Wellness Center
Fort Collins, Colorado

4

Birth
Trauma

"The nervous system is the most complicated and highly
organized of the various systems which make up the
human body. It is the mechanism concerned with
the correlation and integration of various bodily
processes and the reactions and adjustments
of the organism to its environment."

Anatomy of the Human Body
[Gray's Anatomy]
Henry Gray
(1821-1865)

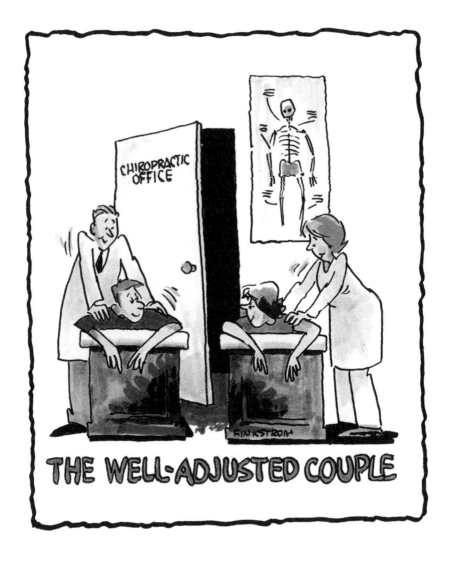

Hospital Rounds

Dr. Monroe Schneier, a chiropractor, and his family had just returned from visiting relatives in New York. It was a Saturday night, and he was tired from the drive. There was a message on his answering machine. It could wait 'til morning. "Oh, what the heck," he thought as he pressed the playback button. Jeff Verbet, a chiropractor in nearby Harrisburg, had called. His voice was very somber. "Monroe, call me as soon as you can." Monroe called immediately.

"Jeff, what's wrong?"

"Cookie (Jeff's wife) just gave birth to a boy this morning, but he isn't expected to live. He can't accept nutrition in any form. They asked permission to do an autopsy tomorrow morning."

"Did you adjust the child?"

"No. That's why I'm calling. Will you?"

"If they'll let me in the hospital, I will!"

"I'll call you right back." Five minutes later, Jeff called. "I told the pediatrician I was having another doctor, a specialist from New York, come in to evaluate my child. He said that would be okay; he'd leave word at the hospital. I gave him your name."

Picture the scene. It's midnight; and two tired men are sitting in the darkened waiting room at Holy Spirit Hospital in Camp Hill, Pennsylvania. A nurse came over: "Dr. Schneier?"

"Yes?"

"We can start now." Both men rose. The nurse turned to the father, "I'm sorry sir; you'll have to wait here."

Dr. Schneier later recalled, "They put a mask on me, a white coat and cap, and led me into the nursery. Soon, the nurse came back with this dried out little bundle. The baby couldn't even cry; he was *trying* to cry, but couldn't make any sound. He was so tiny, just a few hours old. I said to the nurse, 'put the baby on the bassinet.' The nurse did as she was told.

"I turned the baby on his stomach. I did my usual checks and adjusted a couple of dorsal and cervical vertebrae. The nurse's eyes looked like they were going to pop out of her head, but she didn't say anything. I handed the baby back to her. She asked me to fill out a paper with my name, diagnosis, and prognosis. I wrote Monroe Schneier, DC, where I practiced in Middletown, Pennsylvania, and—under diagnosis—wrote, 'Subluxations in the cervical and dorsal spine.' Under prognosis, I wrote, 'Baby will be fine.' I then took off the mask, coat and hat, and walked out.

"I took Jeff to a local watering hole and bought him a drink. He needed it. After that, I went to bed. Between the ride from New York and the newborn adjustment at the hospital, I was exhausted. But first thing next morning, I called Jeff."

"Jeff, how's the baby?"

"Monroe, the baby and Cookie are both home."

"What? Home?"

"In the middle of the night, the baby started to accept nutrition. By morning, he was doing just fine. Cookie got dressed, wrapped up the baby, called me and said, 'Get us out of here!' I brought them home. Monroe, you are in our hearts forever."

"The hospital gave you permission to leave?"

"Who asked for permission?"

If the story were to end there, it would be enough. I view these stories as bittersweet since most babies in hospitals that need Chiropractic care do not receive it. How many remain sick or die for want of an adjustment? There is a postscript to this Chiropractic miracle.

A few months later, Jeff received a new patient. After the consultation, she said, "I want to tell you how sorry I am."

"About what?" asked Dr. Verbet.

"Well, I'm a nurse at Holy Spirit Hospital. I was on night duty that evening. I was so sorry to hear your baby had died."

"What?" Dr. Verbet looked at his new patient carefully. She seemed sane. A thought struck him. "Wait a minute; I'll be right back."

Jeff operates a home-based practice. He ran upstairs and came back down with a gurgling child saying, "Here's the baby that died."

"What? I..., I..., I just don't understand. The next day, the hospital staff told us the baby died the previous night."

Dr. Verbet is not someone to leave stones unturned. He made an appointment with the pediatrician, ostensibly to bring the baby in for a checkup. He greeted the MD with, "Hey, explain this, will you?"

"I don't know, things happen, the baby made a spontaneous improvement."

"What's this about my baby dying? Why did you say the baby died?"

"I don't have an explanation."

"Why didn't you say the baby had an adjustment?"

"I couldn't. The hospital has rules about that sort of thing. If I had known what your doctor was going to do, I would never have allowed him into the hospital."

"*Even though he saved my baby's life?* Even though now, knowing what you know about how a Chiropractic adjustment saved my baby's life, even *now* you regret doing it? This is insanity. We're leaving. Say goodbye to the baby."

Tedd Koren, DC
Founder and President
Koren Publications, Inc.
Hatfield, Pennsylvania

Chiropractic Saves Lives!

After trying to conceive for almost a year, my wife, Nicole, was pregnant with our first and only child. (We didn't know it at the time—the only child part, that is, but you'll understand why when you get to the end of the story.) As you might imagine, we were extremely happy with the news and couldn't wait until the blessed event!

Nicole's pregnancy would go down in the record books as being really easy. She had almost no morning sickness and enjoyed a nearly pain-free nine months.

Then, on March 19, 2007, at 1:00 in the morning, it happened: Nicole's contractions began...our Big Day had finally arrived. We loaded up the car and headed to the birthing center where our midwife was waiting.

By this time, Nicole was experiencing a lot of pain. She wanted to make sure our baby was brought into this world medication-free, so she had chosen to have a natural birth.

Nicole spent the next eighteen hours in hard labor. She eventually opted to get into the tub to relax and prepare for a "water birth." Little did we know that she hadn't quite made it to the halfway point; she still had twenty more hours to go.

At 7:00am the next day, our midwife informed us that the baby was not positioned properly and it was time to drive to the hospital.

After waiting two hours in the hospital "labor room" with ten other women and then waiting another two hours in a "prep room," the obstetricians informed us that our baby's heart rate had increased to 204 beats per minute and that Nicole was running a fever. My wife's water had been broken for more than twenty hours, and she was running a high risk of infection. For the safety of mother and child, an emergency C-section was directed by the attending doctor.

Nicole and I were both scared, but, with a quiet prayer on my lips, I assured her that everything would be alright. I gave her a kiss on the forehead, and she was whisked off to the operating room.

As I waited nervously in the corridor, the attending doctors informed me it would be a two-hour procedure; they'd let me know as soon as it was completed.

At 4:30pm, the doctors came through the waiting room doors and called, "Mr. Burfield, we need to speak with you in private."

I was escorted down the hall to an isolated room. When I walked through the door, the attending doctor greeted me. "Mr. Burfield, please have a seat." I sat down and the doctor resumed: "We ran into serious complications with your wife's delivery, and she has lost a lot of blood. After the first incision, we were unable to move your baby because the child was firmly lodged in your wife's pelvis. In order to make more room for us to work, we performed a second incision: a 'T-Cut.'

"Even with this procedure, your baby was still locked in the pelvis. We had to invert your wife and use the force of gravity to assist in the delivery. It took two doctors pulling on your daughter to dislodge her.

"When we finally got the baby out, she wasn't breathing; it took us 2 minutes and 41 seconds to resuscitate her. Your daughter is severely bruised; the neck muscles on her right side are damaged, and her right arm is completely paralyzed. On the bright side, everyone is okay; mother and child are alive, and you are the father of a baby girl, Baleigh Caroline Burfield."

Don't ever let anyone tell you grown men don't cry. I bawled like a calf in a Texas roping contest!

The damage to Baleigh's neck muscles would later be diagnosed as *torticollis*. It broke my heart to see my little girl like this. I just wanted to take her and Nicole home.

But before I even left the hospital, I phoned my chiropractor. I explained what had happened, and he agreed to meet us there to give Baleigh an adjustment. Within three hours of her first adjustment, our daughter started to move her right arm. Within two days, she had regained full arm function.

The hospital doctors told us it was a "miracle."

I replied, "You're absolutely right! The power that made the body heals the body."

I eventually scheduled an appointment with Dr. Christine Hyman, a certified pediatric chiropractor in the Dallas area. Her specialty: birth trauma!

Over the course of the next twelve months, Baleigh was seen once a week at Dr. Hyman's office. Within eight months, we saw a dramatic difference in our daughter's damaged neck muscles. Within a year, you couldn't even tell she had had a problem.

True healing takes time. True healing is not a quick fix. I wish more people would get that. During the first six months of her healing process, there were days and nights that Baleigh would just cry and cry—obviously in a lot of pain. There were times when even I wasn't sure she'd ever get better. It was on those days that I learned the true meaning of Faith.

My wife and I both kept the Faith and continued to get Baleigh adjusted every week. Eventually, her body healed completely.

Today, our little girl laughs, our little girl plays, our little girl runs, our little girl skips, our little girl jumps and she does *everything* any normal three-year-old little girl does—and more!

Baleigh is a Chiropractic Miracle! Oh, and by the way; she still gets adjusted once every two weeks because it keeps her healthy. I wish more parents would get that.

Chris W. Burfield
Husband, father, and Chiropractic advocate
Unabashed fan of
Christine Hyman, DC
Farmer's Branch, Texas

Failure to Thrive

As I was adjusting one of my regular patients, I sensed that she was preoccupied with something. She had dropped by my office on her way home from picking up her little six-week-old "preemie" granddaughter who had just been released from the hospital.

The baby had been diagnosed with "Failure to Thrive," and had been kept in the Infant ICU since birth. When insurance and family and community funds were exhausted, the doctors told the mother they had done all they could and to take the baby home and enjoy her for the little time she had left to live.

The infant and her mother were in my office waiting for Grandma, so my wife stepped into the reception area and spoke with the baby's mother. When my wife told the mother that she thought I could help the baby, the mother came to the adjusting room and said—in her thick Southern drawl, "Dr. Watson, if yew thank yew 'kin he'p ma baby, I'd be mighty proud fer ya ta try." She placed the infant in my arms, and I laid her on the adjusting table.

The baby weighed only three pounds, and I could almost fit her whole body in my hand. She had a very weak little cry, and, as I examined her, found her tiny little leg-lengths were off by about three-quarters-of-an-inch. Since unequal leg-length is an indicator of nervous system imbalance, I remembered thinking, "Goodness. What would that be in an *adult?*"

As I gently balanced the infant's little nervous system and then handed her back to her mother, I explained that when the child falls asleep, do not be concerned if she sleeps for a *week.* "Just keep her dry and fed—and *let her sleep!*"

Two months later, Grandma returned for a maintenance visit. As I ushered her back to the adjusting room, my eye caught a woman bouncing a happy little, rosy-cheeked baby on her lap.

The baby looked at me with her big, blue eyes, and flashed a bright little smile at me.

When we reached the adjusting room, Grandma asked, "How do you like my little grandbaby?"

I replied, "You know me, I love *all* little babies."

She said, "Dr. Watson, you don't recognize that baby do you? That's the little baby you adjusted two months ago!"

I was astonished! That little girl in my reception room was the same little baby the doctors had sent home from the hospital to die only two months earlier! Grandma then related to me what had happened after they left my office.

She told me that until that day, the baby hadn't slept for more than three minutes at a time, and that she had been unable to keep anything on her stomach. No matter what she had been fed, it had been vomited back up within just a few minutes.

Grandma said that as they got into the car after leaving the office, the mother fed the child a whole ounce of milk on the way home. It was more than the child had ever eaten in her whole short life! They expected her to throw it all back up again, but she didn't. The baby guzzled the milk down as though she hadn't eaten in months—which she hadn't, and, after being burped, she fell asleep in her mother's arms.

Grandma continued, "It's a good thing you told us not to worry if the child slept for a week, because we would have called the emergency room and taken her back to the hospital when she hadn't awakened after 36 hours.

The baby finally awoke just long enough to be fed and changed; then went back to sleep again. Within just a few days, she had regulated to a normal eat-sleep pattern and began to thrive. With her tiny nervous system unlocked, within two month's time she had gained eleven-and-a-half pounds and had grown into the beautiful little fifteen-pound beauty that laughed at me as I greeted her Grandma that day.

As if by reflex, I said, "Thank you Heavenly Father. *You* can take credit for this one. I'll take credit for the next one."

I know my place in the grand scheme of things, and I'm still waiting for one I can take credit for. The family *thinks* it was a miracle; I *know* it was a miracle!

John G. Watson, DC (Retired)
With much-appreciated help from Ramona L. Watson
As presented at the
Palmer College of Chiropractic Homecoming
May 2006

Little Baby Nolan

It has been both a privilege and an honor for me to serve in the Chiropractic profession for 37 years. My journey began in 1973 when destiny called, and I entered the Chiropractic world as an assistant in a Red Bud, Illinois, clinic. There, I was introduced to the powerful principles and practices of this noble profession, as well as to the magnificent power of the nervous system—the Master System—controlling all other systems in our bodies.

My journey continued to Port Huron, Michigan, and on to Lawton, Oklahoma, with my late husband, Dr. Marvin Lepien. He was a true pioneer in Chiropractic, practicing nearly 50 years until his death in 1998. He taught me so much—how brave the old Chiropractic warriors had to have been to overcome the stigma of our profession—to pave the road for all of us to follow!

Over the years, I enjoyed the various stages of my Chiropractic journey as a Chiropractic Assistant (CA), as an office manager, as the wife of a chiropractor, as a student at the Parker College of Chiropractic in Dallas, Texas, as the mother of three Chiropractic students, and—since 1991—as a Doctor of Chiropractic!

It has been fantastic and incredibly rewarding to see lives touched and changed in the Chiropractic offices where I worked during those years, and I could share many stories of healing and miracles that would bring tears to your eyes and melt your heart.

However, the story dearest to me—the one I want to share with you here—is that of little baby Nolan.

Nolan's mother and his older brother were happy patients at my clinic, since older brother was healed from severe reflux and leg cramps after getting adjusted. I treated the mother during her pregnancy with twins, a boy and a girl, and did not see her again until a few months after the children were born. I vividly remember the day she entered my office with her newborns. It was then that she shared her story.

"When the twins were two weeks old, an orthopedic doctor thought that baby Nolan had hip dysplasia and put him in a brace. Then, they noticed that he never turned his head. The medical doctors at the local military base said he had had a "mild stroke" and was therefore unable to move his left side, that he had severe torticollis (twisting of muscles of the neck beyond their normal position), and that he needed surgery. Their next diagnosis was cerebral palsy, and it was suggested that Nolan might need to be placed in an institution since he was never going to be a 'normal' child."

Tears streamed down the face of Nolan's mother as she reached out and handed me her precious little three-month-old.

Please appreciate that I am a confident and positive person with the greatest faith in my Chiropractic skills. But at that moment, as I was entrusted with the life of this little boy, my heart and my thoughts went directly to God in a prayer of petition to give me the insight and guidance to handle this special patient. Following this guidance, while examining Nolan, I concluded that he indeed did not suffer from a stroke, but that his upper cervical spine was injured during the birthing process. From my deep, inner spiritual being, I gently started laying hands on Nolan, adjusting his entire little spine. At the time, he was not able to turn his head on his own, nor was he aware of his surroundings.

My heart leapt for joy when, later that evening, a call came from Nolan's mother. Her son had lifted his head and looked at her for the very first time!

We continued his adjustments on a regular basis for a few weeks with remarkable changes noted on an ongoing basis. After about two months of care, Nolan had caught up with his twin sister and they continued their journey of development and growth together—subluxation free, and in a healthy and normal fashion.

A *miracle* had happened; a life was saved—all due to the power of Chiropractic. By removing the interference at the spinal level caused by birth trauma, the intelligence and the energy of the nervous system was freed to express itself fully and completely in his delicate little body—resulting in normal function and a normal life. Thank God for Chiropractic!

I will continue serving humanity, touching lives, and performing miracles through Chiropractic for the rest of my life.

Rose Lepien, DC
Aaragon Chiropractic Clinic
Lawton, Oklahoma

A Strong Right Arm

When I first saw two-year-old Timmy, he walked into my office with his right arm held tightly against his chest. His grandfather had brought the youngster to see me in the hope I could help the boy. Timmy had no use of his right arm whatsoever; it simply wasn't developing like his left arm.

Grandpa told me that Timmy's mother had had a rough time with labor and, during the boy's delivery, the doctors had found it necessary to use forceps. As a result, the nerves from his neck that controlled his right arm had been damaged. This caused a loss of control of the arm muscles. Timmy's fingers had no sensation of touch, and his right arm was noticeably smaller and shorter than the left.

Timmy never complained about pain or discomfort during our examination; his arm just wouldn't work. The medical doctors had labeled his disability *Erb's Palsy,* or damage to the nerves that run the arm. They told his parents there was nothing more they could do, and that Timmy would have to spend the rest of his life with a crippled arm.

I, too, was concerned that Timmy had sustained permanent, irreversible nerve damage and admitted that I wasn't sure if Chiropractic care would help...but I *was* willing to try! I gave Timmy specific spinal adjustments in the hope they would restore the ability of his nerves to send messages back and forth between his brain and the deformed arm.

As his care progressed, Timmy started to walk with his bad arm hanging at his side instead of held tightly against his chest. His mother was all excited one day when she brought him in for adjustment. She reported that Timmy had reached up with his right hand and turned a door knob!

Soon, he was lying on the floor coloring with crayons and writing with a pencil—activity that made use of his right arm and hand. Power and fine-muscle control was being restored in that disabled arm. One evening, Timmy's parents watched in amazement and delight as their son danced around the family room playing his toy guitar and singing at the top of his lungs: "Doctor Werner healed my arm! Doctor Werner healed my arm!" This news brought tears to my eyes.

Then, I didn't see Timmy for a while. Several years later, when he was eight, his mother brought him in for a check up. He looked and acted like any normal, growing boy. Both arms measured the same length, and he had developed quite a strong grip. He proudly told me he was playing lacrosse and hockey.

"So, what's the message?" you may ask. Simply this: We never should doubt the power of the body and its potential to heal and repair. Here was a little boy who was destined for a life of disability. But, given the proper care and the opportunity, his body was able to recreate a healthy arm when many experts said it could not be done.

William C. Werner, DC
Hagersville Chiropractic
Hagersville, Ontario
CANADA

The Jamie Clark Story

This story demonstrates the positive impact of Chiropractic on human physiology as it relates to children. Please bear in mind that this account comes from an office where all but a few of the 140-plus children formerly seen each week were symptom-free. Of the small number treated that presented with symptoms, the case of Jamie Clark is the most profound I've experienced in my long career. It is my honor and privilege to share her story with you. (To Chiropractic patients and others reading this story, don't let the occasional clinical terminology intimidate you, simply "go with the flow" and accept that the highly-specialized vocabulary used here is common in the healthcare field.)

Jamie Clark was born on February 15, 1993, via modern technological obstetrical procedures. A C-section baby, she experienced severe fetal distress during delivery. Vacuum extraction was used to pull her through the lower abdominal incision. The suction cup left Jamie's face black and blue from the crown of her head to her eyebrows. Within three weeks, the discoloration disappeared, but a large cephalohematoma (bulge on the head due to the accumulation of blood between scalp and skull) remained. Jamie was sent to St. Mary's Hospital in Langhorne, Pennsylvania, for x-rays that revealed a calcified hematoma. Her own body dissolved the calcification within four months and the bulge disappeared.

On April 19, 1993 (two months and four days after birth), Jamie was taken to a pediatrician for a routine checkup. She received the standard DPT (a single, combined vaccine for diphtheria, pertussis, and tetanus) and oral polio vaccines. Within three weeks, Jamie developed an ear infection that was treated with Amoxicillin (an antibiotic) to no avail. A week later, Ceclor (another antibiotic) was prescribed. Jamie started vomiting excessively, refused bottles, became restless, and slept in intervals of no more than two- to three-hours. She developed diarrhea, kicked and stiffened her body, and cried continually.

In early June 1993, Jamie was referred to Philadelphia Children's Hospital. Her baby formula was changed to Nutramigen, a predigested hypoallergenic formula. Every 48 hours, stool hemocultures consistently revealed blood in her feces.

On June 18, 1993, Jamie was given a barium upper gastrointestinal tract examination. The result was negative with no evidence of esophageal reflux. Blood and stool specimens were taken. Blood was still present in the feces. Her gastroenterological diagnosis included post-viral enteritis, C-difficile enteritis, colitis secondary to antibiotic usage, allergic colitis, gastroesophageal reflux with esophagitis (exquisitely nasty heartburn), gastric and/or duodenal ulcer disease, and duodenitis secondary to congenital or autoimmune phenomena.

On June 22, 1993, Jamie received Demerol (a painkiller) and Versed (an anesthetic) by intravenous injection in preparation for an upper endoscopy where a tube was inserted into her mouth, down through her esophagus and stomach, and into her duodenum. As the tube was withdrawn, biopsies were taken from the duodenum, the antrum of the stomach, and the esophagus. Results revealed duodenitis and esophagitis; Zantac (stomach acid production inhibitor) and Reglan (a strong antacid) were prescribed.

On July 9, 1993, a gastric-emptying study, or milk scan, was performed by mixing baby formula with Technetium and sulfur colloid. The results showed no definite evidence of reflux into the upper esophagus, but did reveal a marked delay in the initial rate of stomach emptying. It suggested an antral grinding dysfunction.

On July 15, 1993, at a followup visit with Jamie's pediatrician, DPT, oral polio (second dose), and HIB (Haemophilus Influenza Type B Vaccine) shots were administered. Since the ear infection was still present, SMZ-TMP, another antibiotic, was prescribed. Due to Jamie's apparent club feet, she was referred to an orthopedic surgeon for examination.

On July 19, 1993, the ear infection had progressed to both ears. The pediatrician prescribed Lorabid suspension as a new element in yet another regimen of antibiotics.

On July 21, 1993, the ear infection had worsened and Erythromycin (an antibiotic) was prescribed with the recommendation that inner ear tubes be inserted.

On July 29, 1993, the ear infection finally cleared. The pediatrician suggested Amoxicillin as a prophylactic antibiotic therapy (ongoing for prevention). The parents refused.

On July 30, 1993, the orthopedic surgeon recommended the tearing of Jamie's feet ligaments, corrective casts, and possible Fillauer bars with corrective shoes to deal with Jamie's club feet. Jamie, now five-and-a-half months old, was taking antibiotics three times a day, Zantac twice a day, Reglan four times a day, plus Tylenol and Anbesol. She had become chemically toxic and was facing orthopedic surgery.

On August 4, 1993, (five months and seventeen days after her birth) I saw Jamie Clark for the first time. Her parents reported that she was very irritable, vomited frequently, slept sporadically, and had stomach pain. She was very thin, pale, and lifeless. I held a gentle contact on her left occiput, a double notch contact on her sacrum, adjusted Jamie's right temporal suture (right side of skull) and her atlas vertebra (first vertebrae in the neck). Since I couldn't tell the parents to take her off all medications—that constitutes the practice of medicine, I stated that, if she were my baby, I would take the child off every single drug.

Two days later, Jamie returned to my office a very happy infant. She was sleeping better, eating well, and had no stomach pain. I adjusted her again and placed her on a three-times-a-week Chiropractic care schedule. The parents asked: "What about the bow legs and club feet?" I explained that all I could do was clear the nervous system of interferences caused by subluxations; the rest was up to Jamie's innate ability to heal.

I also explained that I monitor heel tension, foot flare, leg length, leg adduction, ankle flare, microwave emission, and muscle tone as a means of analyzing the neuro-spinal system. I usually notice a reduction in these variables after adjustments. This means that in most people, alignment of the legs, ankles and feet shifts naturally as a result of spinal adjustments. After each visit, Jamie showed dramatic improvement; her legs and feet were turning toward "normal."

A followup visit to the Bucks County Orthopedic Group confirmed that Jamie's hips were indeed normal, her knees were normal, and, although her feet still had a mild metatarsus adductus deformity, I knew from experience that this condition would resolve spontaneously without orthopedic intervention.

It is my firm conviction that Jamie's club feet and bow legs were caused by excessive spinal cord tension due to subluxations produced by a traumatic birth. Her situation was further complicated by chemical overload from numerous medications and by physical stress from the numerous medical procedures.

By the time I left practice in 1997, Jamie, then four years old, was coming in for wellness care on a regular basis along with her parents. She was a completely normal baby—happy, healthy, and walking like any other child her age. I often wonder:

What would have happened to Jamie if she had continued down the medical interventions road?

What would have happened if I had refused to see her because she didn't have back pain or any apparent muscular or skeletal problems?

What would have happened if the neighbors that referred her to my office had believed Chiropractic is only for bad backs?

Would they have talked to Jamie's parents, pleading with them to send her to a chiropractor?

What would have happened if I had played medical doctor and requested all of her medical records, took x-rays, and performed orthopedic and neurological exams prior to adjusting her? Wouldn't I have duplicated the very approach that failed to make her well? Would her parents have allowed it after all they had seen their baby go through? Would they have thought: What a fool I—a "mere" chiropractor—was to attempt to compete with and duplicate the very best medical care a child could get at Philadelphia Children's Hospital?

Instead, I acted in the "Now Moment." My heart was wide open in understanding the plight and suffering of this infant. I acted out of the goodness in my heart, in total trust that within that tiny sick body was trapped a healthy, joyful infant. I used my formal Chiropractic education, coupled with the edge of intuition and instinct honed during two decades of daily practice, letting my senses give me a full reading of Jamie's subluxation pattern. Instead of addressing the darkness and what was *wrong* with her, I turned on the light and addressed what was *right* in her.

To me, Chiropractic is not an alternative to medicine. Chiropractic stands on its own; and everyone can enjoy its benefit, whether sick or well.

Medicine is about *sickness* and *disease*.

Chiropractic is about LIFE!

Arno Burnier, DC
Café of Life
Chiropractic Consulting
Durango, Colorado

5

Pediatric Wellness

"Many things can wait; the child cannot.
Now is the time his bones are being
formed, his mind is being developed.
To him we cannot say tomorrow;
his name is today."

Gabriela Mistral, pen name for
Chilean-born Lucila Godoy y Alcayaga
1945 winner of the Nobel Prize for Literature
(1889-1957)

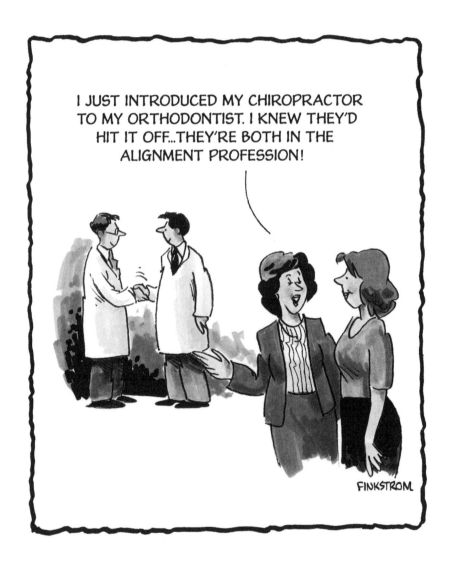

Reprinted by arrangement with Finkstrom Licensing International

In Search of
La Bella Vita
(The Beautiful Life)

"Put your hand on a hot stove for a minute, and it seems like an hour. Sit with a pretty girl for an hour, and it seems like a minute. *That's* relativity."

Albert Einstein

My daughter's name is Isabella. When I speak to my little girl today, it's only natural to reach for the shorter version of her Italian name and just say, "Bella." This, my first child, came into the world with a silky cap of red hair, skin the color of French porcelain, and eyes the shade of a summer sky. If ever a child was born beautiful, Isabella was.

And how delighted I was to be a mother. Like many young women, I had looked forward to loving and being loved by the baby in my arms. Certainly that experience is central to the happiness of a family. But my family's reality abruptly crashed one morning in June as my husband took Bella in his arms, gently bathed her little body in the warm, sudsy water of our kitchen sink, and stroked her shoulders with a tiny washcloth. Suddenly there was a scream. "Jessica! JESSICA!"

I ran from the backyard, tore open the patio door, and found my husband struggling to hold onto Bella as she convulsed in the water. Her little arms and legs had stiffened out straight, and her eyes had rolled up and backwards. A *grand mal* seizure is an ugly thing to see. It's two minutes of terror that nearly stopped my own heart.

That was just the beginning. Our family doctor sent us to a pediatrician who, in turn, referred us to a neurologist. Despite all their efforts, Bella continued to suffer seizures—even as we tried and exhausted a regimen of prescription drugs, clinical exams, and test after test after test. On an almost continuous basis, either Steven or I would be with Bella at the hospital—a "children's hospital" filled with patients afflicted like Bella, or worse. With each passing day—and with every conflicting diagnosis, our daughter's condition grew increasingly grave while my husband and I became increasingly more desperate.

Even in the most loving of families, chronic illness in one individual spreads emotionally throughout the household. When you're force-fed a diet of anxiety and fear, the tension between husband and wife becomes like a persistent bad taste in your mouth. Denying or ignoring that effect is hazardous to your marriage; and it threatens the well-being of everyone in your home—including that of the patient. Our family was no exception. Somehow, Steven and I got through those first challenging days, with months and years of Bella's illness yet to come. But as anyone with a seriously-ill child can tell you, it takes more than love for a family to endure these things. You have to summon up every shred of fortitude in your heart to survive and come out whole.

Medically, there were no consistent answers for Bella. We plodded on as best we could. As we anticipated our firstborn's second birthday, I discovered that I was once-again pregnant. In 2005, Nicolas was born. How thrilled we were to have both a daughter and now a son. Like his sister, our baby boy was incredibly beautiful. But our pure delight soon faded. Nicolas developed respiratory problems, was re-admitted to the hospital, and thus began *his* trials and tribulations. Just when you think nothing can break you, life heaps on more adversity. On some days, I simply told myself, "Keep breathing. This, too, shall pass." I'm no saint. But I do believe that things happen for a reason and that God allows the testing of our souls—and the blessing of our lives.

Dante was born in 2007. A strong, happy baby, he completed our family and brought us great joy. As a family of five, we continued as before, seeking answers for the problems Bella and Nicolas faced day after day. I have to confess that there were evenings when we resorted to a time-tested strategy used by parents around the globe. I stand amazed at the wonder of the automobile and its reliable ability to lull a baby to sleep! Steven and I buckle the children into their car seats, strap ourselves in, and drive off down the road for a brief cruise. The children fall asleep while Mom and Dad enjoy a bit of quiet time to themselves. It works for us, even as it demonstrates my personal philosophy of parenting: do whatever works for you.

Speaking of things that work for you, it's time for me to reveal how this story ends—or rather, how our lives had a new beginning. On one of our daytime drives, Steven and I spotted a sign posted on the lawn of a neighborhood school, "Kid's Day International." We didn't know what that day involved, but something told us to stop. And how glad I am that we did. In the school gymnasium, a colorful fair was set up, complete with informational booths about children's health. That's where and when we met Dr. David Covey from New Freedom Chiropractic. In a rush of words, Steven and I shared a bit of our story. As we blurted out phrases, Dr. Covey completed our sentences. Before we had a chance to explain, he grasped completely what Bella and Nicolas were suffering. Scans of the children's spines were made right there—on the spot—and revealed that they both had serious alignment problems. Dr. Covey told us that spinal alignment problems are what chiropractors spend years in college learning how to correct. So, as we continued to talk, I felt the first flickers of real hope start to rise in my heart.

Those hopes were not in vain. Starting on that nightmarish June morning when Steven was bathing Bella in the kitchen sink—and up until she began Chiropractic care with Dr. Covey—our daughter had suffered an average of *six seizures a day!* Almost immediately after her first adjustment, a *new* Bella—a Bella that Steven and I had never seen before—miraculously began to emerge. With the healing made possible by Chiropractic care, we were able to wean her off narcotic medications, even as her seizures decreased in length and severity. Gone was her dull, drug-induced listlessness; Bella greeted each successive day with increasing energy and irrepressible enthusiasm.

It wasn't long afterward that Dr. Covey began treating Nicolas. Today, our little boy is flourishing too—his chronic lung infections are gone *for good*—and he's better able to enjoy playing with his older, healthier sister and baby brother. "And where is their favorite place to play?" you might ask. "On *summer camping trips,* that's where!" Just as illness brings suffering to an entire household, so too does health bring a rosier glow to the cheeks of every family member. One look at Bella is proof enough.

The little red-haired doll I first beheld seven years ago is a heartbreaker today. Soft curls frame Bella's face and drift across her forehead. The blue eyes she was born with have deepened into the most beguiling shade of hazel-green. She is ever more a beauty. And like all legendary beauties, Bella knows how to dress. Just this morning she snugged her great-great-grandmother's flower bedecked hat down on her too-small head, then pulled a flaming red plaid dress overtop of her bright pink tights. She draped a cascade of iridescent purple beads across the bodice of the dress, then grabbed a star-emblazoned black scarf, wrapped it around her neck and—with a little help from Mom—casually tied the ends into a stylish bow. Because no trendsetter would be caught dead without drop-dead-gorgeous shoes, Bella chose well: hi-top "tennies," size 1, in blue canvas printed with red roses. You see? From head to toe, my daughter is more than beautiful, she's adorable.

Today, Bella has what I've always wanted for her—a beautiful life. For that, I thank God above; and I thank Dr. Covey.

In my nightly prayers of thanksgiving, I never forget to ask God that, some day, *each and every one* of the little patients in those "children's hospitals" all over the world might also enjoy a beautiful life—through the blessing of Chiropractic!

Jessica Crocker-Idone
Chiropractic advocate
Mother of Isabella Idone,
A happy, healthy patient of
David Covey, DC
New Freedom Chiropractic
Orleans, Ontario
CANADA
As told to Scherry Cooley

Happiness Is a Little Heart

Julie's heart was filled with apprehension the first day she brought her little boy to our office. Could she dare hope that *a chiropractor* was someone that could finally give her son relief?

Since infancy, Cole's two-and-a-half years had been filled with chronic coughing, congestion, wheezing, and ear infections. All 27 pounds of him wished that he could run, wrestle, and play with Brady, his older brother. Sadly, Cole just didn't have enough energy for these normal childhood activities. In fact, a mere few minutes of play would leave him completely exhausted and gasping for breath. Would Cole ever know how much fun it is to play in the snow? Would he ever build a snowman and place a top hat on his winter creation? Would he ever ride a bike like other kids, or build a sand castle at the beach? Would this boy ever run through a field of springtime wildflowers with a new puppy nipping at his heels? Not unless a miracle happened!

Cole's daycare provider was one of our patients. She suggested to Julie and Kurt, Cole's parents, that they consider Chiropractic treatment as a new avenue of care. "What do you have to lose?" she asked. "No one has helped Cole so far; and extensive, around-the-clock medication is obviously causing him severe side effects. Just give Chiropractic a try!"

Cole's health issues weighed heavily on his parents, his brother, and his daycare provider. Being on the front line, so-to-speak, Cole's daycare provider could see that this little boy's energy resources were practically non-existent. Of course, the fact that he had no appetite meant he had no nutrition with which to fuel his energy needs! It's no surprise that the frequency of his bowel movements was about once every five days. (Nothing in means nothing out—that's how the alimentary canal works!) Everyone agreed: the time had come to make a change in Cole's healthcare modality.

On the way to our office, Julie's thoughts reflected back to Cole's infancy. At the age of nine months, he had suffered with pneumonia, a double-ear infection, croup, and dehydration. When he reached one-and-a-half years of age, he had had to endure a tympanoplasty (ear-tube surgery). His frequent attacks of asthmatic bronchitis—and the dangerous breathing difficulties these episodes produced—warranted many anxiety-filled trips to the emergency room. Julie, a nurse by profession, felt utterly helpless as she watched her son suffer.

As she pulled into our clinic parking lot, Julie's medically-inspired doubts about the effectiveness of Chiropractic nagged at her. "How can this possibly help?" she wondered. "Don't chiropractors only adjust backs and necks?" That was what she had been led to believe in her nursing school curriculum. She looked into Cole's big, sunken brown eyes—now outlined by dark circles—and said, "Sweetie, I brought you here to see a new doctor. He's going to try and make you better without pills." Cole clutched his favorite stuffed animal as his mother stood at the doorway of our clinic. At that moment, Julie and her son had no way of knowing they were on the threshold of a new beginning!

Cole and Julie were greeted warmly by our receptionist. After being ushered into an exam room, Julie related the extensive history of a little boy whose memories were not happy ones of running and playing with friends. Instead, they were scary ones of going to medical doctors, hospitals, and emergency rooms. Our doctor listened with great empathy to the pain and frustration in Julie's voice and vowed he would do everything possible to help this little boy with the big, brown, *sad* eyes.

After a thorough exam, the time arrived for Cole's first adjustment. Not knowing what to expect, this brave little soul laid on the chiropractic table with his mom standing at his side. Because pain and suffering had been the major part of his life, Cole showed no fear and never shed a tear. During this brave child's treatment, the only visible reaction was that he winced a couple of times. When the adjustments were finished, Julie scheduled another appointment for the next day in the desperate hope that this new option of care would make a difference.

When they arrived for Cole's second appointment, there was a glimmer of hope in Julie's voice as she said, "Is it possible these treatments are really going to help? Cole took a nap after his adjustment yesterday, and I had to wake him up. For the first time in his life, he slept through the night!" The excitement and optimism in Julie's voice was palpable!

Cole was not the least bit apprehensive about getting on the table for his second adjustment. By his third appointment, Julie reported that Cole's coughing and wheezing had begun to subside. As he progressed in his treatment plan, his overall health improved steadily. "Amazing!" was the only word Cole's daycare provider could use to describe the change in Cole's stamina. He was playing without getting fatigued. He developed an appetite, and was gaining weight. His bowel movements became normal, and he was sleeping all night.

Initially, we saw Cole at the rate of three times a week. Just two months later, we were seeing him just once every two weeks. He continues to gain weight and is off all medications. There are no signs of wheezing or coughing; and he has boundless positive energy. He loves his adjustments and climbs right up on the table when he comes into the clinic. He always has a big smile for everyone and the dark circles are gone from his eyes.

Cole's parents say that all their energy prior to Chiropractic care revolved around his sickness and trying to get him to a comfort level they could all deal with. Now, that same energy is still high, but has changed to the positive field with them trying to keep up with their happy, healthy, *energetic* little boy who finally has a big brother that can't wait to play with him.

The last time we saw Cole at our clinic, he was excited because he had brought a gift for his new best friend, his chiropractor! He had an envelope in his hand, and being very shy, hesitated to give it to the doctor. Finally, without a word, his hand shot out and he handed it over. The doctor accepted the offering with gratitude, looked down, and saw that Cole had traced the outline of his little hand on the back of the envelope. Inside was a *homemade* card—*the very best kind of card*—that read as follows:

> "You brought a gift of kindness
> To a lucky little kid.
>
> "A little life was nurtured
> By all you said and did.
>
> "A little heart felt happy;
> A little person grew.
>
> "A little one was loved
> A whole lot more—because of you!

The envelope also contained a short note:

> We all want to say thank you for helping Cole feel so much better. Words alone cannot tell you how much your care has meant to our family! We now have a healthy little guy that is full of life and feeling great!
>
> Thank you so much,
>
> *Kurt, Julie, Brady, and Cole*

Martin Furlong, DC
MetroEast Wellness Center
Written by Pat Coffey, CA
Cottage Grove, Minnesota

Bright-Eyed, Sleepy Baby

One of my favorite experiences in practice has been repeated numerous times—treating the colic baby. Most people know it's tough to be with a screaming infant that seemingly refuses to be consoled. The situation is made worse since "baby" can't communicate what's wrong. Finding it impossible to calm their child, caring parents are often torn by feelings of helplessness. At the same time, they're being driven crazy by the noise!

One particular infant had been unmercifully poked and prodded by medical doctors for the first three months of his life. Unable to properly diagnose the boy's problem, the medical world dismissed him as nothing more than a "fussy baby." Through friends, the parents of this child had heard that Chiropractic might be helpful and were referred to my practice.

After a detailed examination, I concluded that this poor little guy may have been suffering with severe headaches since birth. The cause: his first two vertebrae, the atlas and axis, were misaligned during the delivery process. I then checked a series of other details including his digestive system, which had not been working very well either. Next, I reviewed the previous lab results and other diagnostics prescribed by the medical world— the main focus of the infant's medical doctors. The final, pretreatment analysis involved a review of the medical and alternative procedures previously administered along with a full range of questions about his diet. Now, with the preliminaries taken care of, it was time for our new patient's Chiropractic treatment.

This screaming infant's first adjustment was a "diversified alignment" of the first two vertebrae which he tolerated very well.

In fact, immediately after the adjustment, his crying stopped and his eyes opened wide to see what had just removed that terrible pressure from inside his head. He then sucked in a huge breath of fresh air and—obviously exhausted from sleep deprivation—immediately relaxed into a nice nap. All of this happened within about four-to-five minutes. Standing by my side during the procedure, the boy's mother was so happy on seeing this great miracle she broke down into joyful tears. The father appeared awestruck by what he had witnessed.

The next morning, having had the first full night's sleep since her son's birth—another miracle as far as she was concerned, the patient's mother called to express her thanks. After a few additional adjustments with a little tummy work and some digestive enzymes, this little guy was transformed into a happy, healthy, baby boy. It gives me enormous pleasure to report that this young man has matured into a strong athlete who is still getting regular adjustments to keep his sporting life as active as possible.

As mentioned earlier, I've been blessed with the opportunity to successfully treat colic babies numerous times in my career. The stories are too many to count of how my patients in all age groups have benefitted from an immediate "miracle treatment" releasing things from ear infections, sight problems, to even complicated cases of cancer and chronic disease. These results clearly show the power of Chiropractic to release the powerful energy flow that God has put within us. The daily opportunity to observe the effectiveness of this healing art inspires us physicians in our efforts to make Chiropractic the world's number one healthcare modality. I've been blessed myself with regular adjustments since I was just a few days old. Now, well into my forties, I've had no immunizations or antibiotics—ever! The power of Chiropractic never ceases to amaze me; and I see miracles happen every day!

Dave Jensen, DC, CCSP, DACBSP
WIN Health Institute
Aspen, Colorado

I Love You, Mommy

I cannot tell this story enough. For us, Chiropractic has been the answer to a serious problem.

My husband and I were experiencing severe tantrums with Zachary, one of our two-and-a-half-year-old twins. The pediatrician said our distressed son was normal—but at the "extreme end of the behavior scale." As Zach's mother, I wasn't satisfied with that answer. I felt he was acutely uncomfortable—in some kind of pain, and I was desperately searching for answers.

Zachary's tantrums sometimes lasted as long as an hour. They included sobbing, nonsense babbling, throwing and breaking things, and often hurting himself: whether biting his flesh, pulling his hair, or hitting his own head. He'd just lose control and throw himself down *anywhere*: once, down a concrete staircase onto a concrete patio; often, in the middle of the street. Sometimes, he'd repeat, "*Help me! Help me! Help me!*" Almost *anything* could spark the tantrums—just a noise or sound he didn't like would set him off. He could be seized by as many as five-to-six hour-long tantrums in a single day.

The behavior started when Zach was little more than a year old and got progressively worse from there on. His communication skills—which, to our delight, had developed early—regressed, to our obvious dismay. Instead of exchanging information in typical toddler conversation, he often simply repeated the question asked—or other words said to him. He usually preferred to sit alone rather than have someone sit next to him.

We put Zach on a special diet that excluded sugar, wheat, dairy, and more. We eliminated many cleaning chemicals and perfumes from our home fearing chemical sensitivity. While these steps yielded *some* improvements, they were not enough to make life with a *normal* six-year-old, a *normal* two-and-a-half-year-old, and an *out-of-control* two-and-a-half-year-old manageable.

Zach's destructive behavior took its toll on our entire family.

I had every reason to fear that Zachary, or I, or *both* of us would soon need to be medicated. The truth is that *I* was on the verge of a nervous breakdown; I was afraid to leave the house with Zach, and I was crying all the time. Finally, my husband relented and allowed me to take our troubled son to my chiropractor—we needed a *miracle!* (Although I've been under Chiropractic care regularly since I was 15, my husband initially was opposed to non-medical treatment for our children.) My goal was to relieve whatever it was that was causing Zach discomfort so that his tantrums would become more manageable.

Under steady Chiropractic care, we immediately saw a reduction in the *severity* of the tantrums although the *frequency* was initially unchanged. After five weeks of regular visits, however, the results have been nothing short of miraculous.

The tantrums have become much less frequent and, when they do occur, the episodes last just five-to-ten minutes. Zachary's grandparents commented that they could see that he sometimes makes a conscious effort for control—and often wins the battle! More and more frequently, we can reason him out of a tantrum, and can work with him to "stay calm." *But there's more!*

Zach's communication skills are back to normal for his age. He again initiates conversations, comments reasonably on things, and asks and responds to questions. But perhaps my favorite improvement is the emotional one. He sits with me often and gives me as many kisses and hugs as I ask for. He says, "*I love you, Mommy!*" whenever the feeling strikes him. I couldn't be happier.

Some people are skeptical that Chiropractic was the answer. They say Zachary simply outgrew the old behavior pattern. I might agree, *except* for the fact that the improvement has been *sudden* and *three-fold*. His behavior, communication, and emotional responses have *all* improved drastically. More compelling is the fact that these improvements coincide perfectly with Zach's visits to our chiropractor. Quite simply, these improvements have been *everything* my husband and I could possibly have hoped for!

Susan D. Boerchers, freelance writer,
Wife, mother, and Chiropractic advocate
Mother of Zachary Boerchers
A happy, healthy patient of
Gregory R. Salmond, DC
Salmond Family Chiropractic
Flanders, New Jersey

Adapted from an article in
Pathways to Family Wellness magazine
Published by the
International Chiropractic Pediatric Association

Good Tidings from Singapore

To Whom It May Concern:

First of all, I am so glad to know Dr. Curry Wong. She helped me to understand Chiropractic, as it is totally new to me. In the past, I thought Chiropractic was only for people who sprained or strained their low back. I have never thought that Chiropractic could help in many different conditions until her explanations about Chiropractic. Surprisingly to me, even newborns, infants, and older children can also benefit from Chiropractic. Her explanations helped me to have a deeper understanding and changed my impression about Chiropractic. She is the first chiropractor whom I know who specializes in Chiropractic pediatrics. I greatly appreciated her tender and loving care for my baby girl as she received her very first Chiropractic adjustment ever.

I have a very deep impression about that amazing Chiropractic adjustment. When my baby girl was nine-months old, she was teething and had her first fever. She cried most of the time throughout the day. Being a first-time mother,

I did not know what I could do to make her feel better. Fortuitously, Dr. Wong visited my home and found out that my baby girl was sick. She asked my permission to give my baby girl a Chiropractic check up. Since there was nothing much that I could do, I thought, "Why not give Chiropractic a try?" even though Chiropractic for a baby was totally new to me. Dr. Wong was very patient and provided the Chiropractic check up and adjustment with loving care to my sick girl.

It was the first time that I watched a Chiropractic adjustment being done on an infant. I never thought it could be so quick, simple, and wonderful. Dr. Wong examined my girl's head, neck, and back within a few minutes; then the adjustment was done. A while after the adjustment, I found my girl repeatedly releasing a lot of gas and those were big and loud. I have never found her releasing so much gas. That night, my girl's fever was gone.

It is so amazing how gentle Chiropractic can be for kids and how the adjustment is so soft that it would not frighten the kids, unlike the medical or acupuncture which are more invasive and children are usually frightened of being in the medical clinic. Dr. Wong explained that when the spine and the nervous system are out of balance, the body will react to the imbalances, causing the onset of different conditions. It is important to bring the spinal structure and the body back to balance in order to allow the nervous system to function at the optimal state. This will allow the body to function normally again. This was what happened to my baby girl.

From this great experience, I realized that a healthy spine and the nervous system are very important. I would definitely consult Chiropractic if my precious baby girl is ever sick again because it is so natural and non-invasive. Chiropractic is very suitable for children.

Po Yin Chan
Mother of a baby girl who is
A very happy patient of
Curry Y. L. Wong, DC, CACCP
LGS International Chiropractic
The Adelphi
SINGAPORE

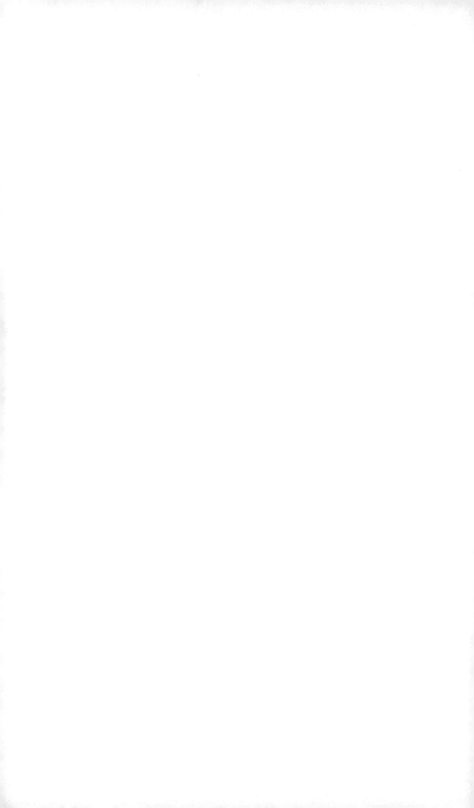

6

Coping with Life's Challenges

"I know God will not give me anything I can't handle.
I just wish that He didn't trust me so much."

Mother Teresa
Albanian-born Agnes Gonxha Bojaxhiu
1979 Nobel Peace Prize winner
Beatified by Pope John Paul II as
Blessed Teresa of Calcutta
after her death
(1910-1997)

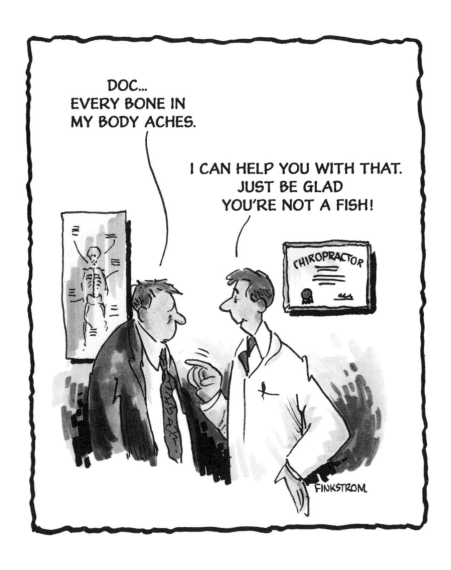

Precious Julia

At nine months into my second pregnancy, "baby" wasn't as eager to greet the world as I was to assist with her timely debut. Seven days later, after fetal monitoring and ultrasound exams, my doctor assured me that everything was quite normal.

At ten days overdue, I returned to the hospital where labor was induced using a cervical gel. Several hours later—around two the next morning—our sweet new baby girl was born. Counting husband David, daughter Rebekah, and me, Julia's arrival made us a cozy foursome.

When Julia was presented to me in the delivery room, I noticed that her entire head was quite bruised. That certainly hadn't been the case when Rebekah was born! I asked myself, "Could I have 'pushed' too hard during labor?" After all, this had been a swift, "natural," pain medication-free delivery. The doctors pointed out that—since Julia's Apgar scores (neonatal test results) were in the normal range—we had nothing to fear.

When we returned home, Julia settled into a baby-blue bassinet adorned with lacy trim and filled with a small menagerie of stuffed animals. Rebekah, now Julia's "big sister," was thrilled to finally welcome her long-awaited sibling.

Julia proved to be an extraordinary baby; she rarely cried. In fact, she only cried about six times in her entire first month. My new daughter was also a very *sleepy* baby. To keep her awake for feedings, I'd have to play with her toes or wipe her face with a damp cloth. In my nursing-mother euphoria, I didn't realize that something was *very* wrong.

At around three weeks, Julia developed her first cold. I thought it a bit unusual because I was breastfeeding her exclusively. Furthermore, she hadn't been around any sickness that I knew of. Unfortunately, this turned out to be the first of many respiratory infections—one about every six-to-eight weeks—for the next *two years!*

Julia's recurring respiratory infections frequently turned into life-threatening ordeals with 911 calls, late-night trips to the ER, and/or multi-day hospitalizations. During these episodes, Julia's airway would swell to the point of her struggling for every breath. Numerous drugs were administered to keep her from choking. We often had to treat her at home with a nebulizer. In the hospital, powerful oral steroids were used to reduce airway inflammation. We often questioned ourselves for giving—and allowing her to be given—so many medications, but felt we simply had no choice.

As the months passed, Julia did not become stronger. She had great difficulty holding her head up if pulled from a lying to a sitting position. She wasn't able to support any weight on her legs. If I lifted her under the arms, it felt as though she could slide through my fingers like a floppy rag doll. I asked my doctor about this, and she simply noted that Julia had poor muscle tone. "Every baby develops at her own pace; Julia will 'catch up' in time," she said. Unsatisfied with this prognosis, I insisted on seeing a specialist and was given an appointment late on a Friday afternoon. After a brief preliminary exam, the pediatrician scheduled a more comprehensive consultation at the hospital the following Monday.

Unwilling to spend the weekend worrying helplessly, I racked my brain for an alternative. Then I remembered seeing a chiropractor recently for my own back pain. With nothing to lose, I called the office first thing Saturday. Surprisingly, they agreed to see Julia right away. Not only did the chiropractor examine and adjust Julia, we received extremely useful information about subluxations and how seriously they can affect one's health. Julia was found to have *severe* upper neck subluxations caused—in all probability—by birth trauma.

At the hospital on Monday, we were assigned to a private consultation room where various specialists took turns visiting us. The pediatrician we had seen Friday was the first to call. Amazingly, when he stood Julia up, there was a brief-but-magical, lifetime-first moment when she held some weight on her legs. Looking back, I'm certain the previous Saturday's Chiropractic adjustment had opened up channels for the right messages to get to the right locations. Julia had *never* stood before.

As Monday's exam continued, we were asked myriad questions regarding family and pregnancy history, if our other child was healthy, etc. We were even asked if my husband and I were possibly *related!* Tests were performed on Julia to study head lag, floppiness, sight, hearing, responsiveness, reflexes, etc. The exam concluded with blood being drawn to check for such conditions as Praeder-Willie Syndrome and Spinal Muscular Atrophy.

When all the results were in, Julia was diagnosed with *central benign hypotonia* (mild central nervous system dysfunction) with no as-yet-discovered cause. Physiotherapy was prescribed through the Infant Development Program of Vancouver; and we continued her Chiropractic care about once every month—we still didn't appreciate the benefits of more frequent Chiropractic treatment.

Julia reached her developmental milestones much later than an average child. She didn't begin to sit on her own until fifteen months. In the nineteen months before learning to crawl, she got around the house by rolling on the floor. Walking was something we thought she might *never* achieve. It wasn't until she was almost two that she could pull herself to a standing position.

In the midst of all this, my pastor-husband was called to start a new church in Toronto, so we had to leave Vancouver. As soon as we settled into our new home, we searched for a chiropractor. At two-and-a-half, Julia was still not walking and was quite weak after recovering from her latest respiratory infection. We had no idea if she would *ever* be well and prayed that God would guide us to a doctor who could give our child the care she so desperately needed.

We soon discovered Inside Out Family Chiropractic—*the answer to our prayers!* When we met Dr. Ryan French, we were overwhelmed by his compassion and concern—not just for Julia, but also for the health of our whole family. At our first guest lecture, we sat in near awe as he explained how even the slightest subluxation can cause major health problems. As I recall sitting in the office waiting for our first Dr. Ryan consultation, I thought, maybe, *just maybe*, we had found the answer for our baby.

Accustomed as we were to Julia's respiratory infections, we weren't surprised when she experienced another episode just a few weeks after starting treatment at Inside Out. *Remarkably, that was her last episode requiring medical intervention!* The frequency of Julia's respiratory problems has dropped dramatically. Now, when she *does* have an infection, her steadily-improving immune system is able to fight it *without the need for pharmaceuticals!*

Imagine our delight when, after just three months of Inside Out care, Julia took her first step. She has since "taken off," and walks short distances unaided, albeit with a stiff gait since she doesn't yet bend her knees. That will surely disappear as her muscle tone improves.

We're certain that the progress we're seeing in Julia is a direct result of the Chiropractic care she's received this past year. The change is so dramatic it's hard to believe she's the same little girl. Holding daddy or mommy's hand, this sick, tired, weak child that we carried into the office almost twelve months ago now walks in and offers a bright smile and a "hello" to everyone. Today, having seen Julia's progress, our entire family enjoys the health-giving benefits of regular adjustments from Dr. Ryan and his Inside Out team.

Epilogue

Just as the arrival of a newborn provides cause for family celebration, the same may be said of weddings. Several months ago, my sister Beth married Johnny Yeomans in a formal-dress ceremony. Early on, Beth asked if Julia could be included in the wedding party. Uncertain as to whether my daughter would be able to walk on cue, we even discussed pulling her down the aisle in a wagon. Ultimately, that idea was abandoned in the fervent hope that Julia would be able to walk.

At the wedding, Julia was dressed and ready—we thought—to serve as one of seven flower girls. Although she managed to make it to the beginning of the aisle with a slow, stiff gait, she changed her mind at the last moment and retreated into the arms of her beloved Great Aunt Melodie—"Auntie" in Julia's list of friends.

The gala reception, however, was another story. With 200 guests seated in the ballroom, proceedings got underway when the master of ceremonies introduced the best man and maid-of-honor. The massive doors at the back of the hall swung open, the couple entered to enthusiastic applause, and the doors were closed again. The cycle was repeated for each pair of bridesmaids and grooms-men followed by the introduction of a sole junior bridesmaid.

The next-to-last group—just ahead of the bride and groom—was the flower girls, adorable young ladies wearing white dresses adorned with yellow satin sashes. Steadied by the hands of Abigail Michel, a friend of the bride, on the left and big sister Rebekah on the right, our precious Julia was greeted by the warm applause of hundreds as she slowly made her *formal* "walking debut." David and I could not hold back the tears.

Elisabeth Wiebe, wife and Chiropractic advocate
Mother of Julia Wiebe, a happy, healthy patient of
Ryan French, DC
Inside Out Family Chiropractic
Bolton, Ontario
CANADA
with Don Dible

Blair's New Report Card

Sister Doreen, one of my regular patients, was a highly-respected and much-revered fifth-grade teacher at a nearby Catholic school in a small Minnesota town. One day, while in my office for a maintenance adjustment, she asked if I could schedule a short presentation on anatomy as part of her class science project the following week. I was more than happy to accept the invitation.

On the Big Day, I brought along a skeleton to use as a prop. When I stood "Mr. Bones" up on the teacher's desk, a hush fell over the class as they studied the display. There was a noticeable movement as each of the children—with no prompting—adjusted from a typical "student slouch" to perfect posture in emulation of Mr. Bones' example!

Before starting my presentation, I looked around and observed that all the students *except one* were seated facing the front-of-the-room chalkboard. Occupying a *separate* desk and chair—at right angles to the rest of the class and against the chalkboard wall—was a very tall young man. (I'd later learn that his name was Blair.) I had no idea why this boy was isolated from the rest of the students; I figured he just needed a "Time Out."

As I delivered my presentation, you could have heard a pin drop whenever I paused for breath. Clearly, Mr. Bones was the focus of everyone's attention. When I finished the lecture, I opened the floor to questions. Almost all of the children eagerly raised their hands in the hope of gaining more insight.

It wasn't until several moments passed that Blair suddenly raised his hand. When I turned and called on him, he reacted as if stunned by my attention. Then, his face quickly transformed into a blank look. His eyes glazed over. His mouth dropped open. And—for what seemed like an eternity—he just stared in my direction. Finally, Blair dropped his arm, and—as he did so— eased his chin to his chest. He slowly shook his head back and forth while mumbling to himself in apparent disappointment.

I wasn't really sure what had happened. I still didn't know why he had been separated from the rest of the class. All I knew was that something wasn't right. So what was wrong? At that point, I wondered if Blair was on drugs (prescription or otherwise), mentally challenged, or both! It didn't really matter to me which, because—just to show you how we chiropractors think— the next question that popped into my mind was: "I wonder what his *spine* looks like?"

I didn't say anything to Blair about my thoughts. Nor did I mention my thoughts to Sister Doreen. I just happen to be one of those people who believe that—if you think about a question long enough and hard enough—an answer will manifest itself. Therefore, you shouldn't be surprised when I tell you who showed up at my clinic three days later.

I had just finished adjusting a patient when I noticed Blair and his mother—she was already a patient of mine—at the front desk. I walked over, said, "Hi!" and asked what had brought them to the office. She told me Blair had epilepsy and that she wanted me to examine him. When I asked why she brought him to see me, a chiropractor, she told me that a friend in Colorado had taken his epileptic daughter to see a chiropractor and that she stopped having seizures. Not surprisingly, Blair's mother wanted the same result for her son.

After filling in Blair's health history, mother and son were shown to a room where I could complete my examination. His mother told me he was suffering as many as eleven "silent seizures" a day. During the seizures, he would, "just go blank!"—a symptom I'd observed during my fifth-grade "Bone Talk." Blair was on two very strong anti-seizure prescription medications. Obviously, they weren't working! Every joint in his body hurt: his knees, ankles, lower back, middle back, neck... *everything!* He was a tall young man—at least six inches taller, and much stronger, than the rest of the kids in his class. He walked very stiff-legged with little bend in his knees. The kids often teased him and called him "Herman Munster!" With so much ribbing, there were times when his frustrations got the best of him. He'd lash out at his classmates...beat on them...and had to be separated from the rest. (That answered my question about his isolated seating in the classroom!) He wet the bed every night, was in a remedial reading class, and consistently brought home report cards featuring D's and F's. How's that for the life of a fifth-grader?

During my examination, I made several abnormal findings. The most significant: Blair had subluxations throughout his spine. Of the 24 moveable segments, 22 were "stuck"...subluxated!

The next day, after studying the rest of Blair's examination report and x-rays, I sat down with him and his mother. I laid out a treatment plan that required adjustments every day for two weeks, three times a week for one month, twice a week for one month, and then once a week for several months thereafter. I presented this long, drawn out treatment plan because Blair needed a lot of work.

His mother accepted my recommendations, and we began adjustments immediately. Six weeks later, we performed a progress examination. Here is what we found:

Blair's joint pain had significantly subsided. By then it was November—the start of basketball season. Since his joints were no longer hurting, Blair went out for the sport. Being by far the tallest kid in his class, he could hold the ball above his head and *nobody* could even get close to stealing it. His popularity grew instantly. Instead of having eleven seizures a day, he was having just one *every other day!* The powerful anti-seizure medication he'd been taking was reduced to just twenty-five percent of the "start-of-Chiropractic-treatment" level. He wasn't wetting the bed anymore and "graduated" from remedial reading class. As his mother gave me his report card, she cried.... Blair was now getting nothing but A's and B's!

If I was a chiropractor who worried about what other people thought of me and only treated neck and back pain, I *never* would have accepted Blair as a patient. After all, you mean: "Chiropractic can help *seizures?*" Blair's results speak for themselves!

Because I believe that you're always better off with a bone *in* place than *out*, I DID treat Blair. It changed his life.... Funny thing is...*he forever changed* my *life!*

David B. Neubauer, DC
Practice Management Consultant
Health Source Chiropractic and Progressive Rehab

Daddy, Daddy, I Love You!

Christopher's mother attended a lecture given by a chiropractor-colleague of mine. He concluded his talk by saying, "I'd like to give each of you a gift—the most precious gift I could ever give anyone. That's the chance for each of you here tonight to give a free Chiropractic checkup to someone you love. I'm not saying I can help. All I'm saying is that it's worth it to find out."

So little Christopher's mother went up to the doctor and said, "My son is autistic; have you ever worked on an autistic child?

"To be honest, I never have, but I can tell you this; a malfunctioning nervous system will destroy your health. And I'd like the chance to find out if Chiropractic care can make a difference for him."

So Christopher's mother brought him in for a Chiropractic assessment. After the boy's third adjustment, the doctor asked his mother to write him a testimonial letter.

She wrote, "My son, Christopher, is six-years old and he's autistic. Christopher has been adjusted just three times by our chiropractor, and I've seen an amazing difference. I noticed Christopher playing less on the computer at home and spending more time interacting on a one-on-one basis with other people.

Christopher's aide and teacher at school mentioned that he was more focused this week, and was less irritable. His printing and coloring have shown marked improvement. His teacher is quite unaware of the Chiropractic care he is receiving."

His mother went on to say that Christopher usually gets somewhere between 60 and 80% on his spelling tests. For the first time in his life, after three adjustments, he got a 100 this week.

But, you know what? That's not where the story ends.

Christopher's father works overseas; and his dad came home for Christmas. He was expecting his son to greet him at the airport the way Christopher had met him his entire life—looking down at the ground and just shaking his head. You see, Christopher had never, ever, looked his dad in the eyes.

This time, Christopher ran toward his father with his head held high and looked his dad squarely in the face. Christopher's father's heart broke when his son opened his mouth and said, "Daddy, daddy, I love you!"

Chiropractors can change the world. If all each of us ever did in our entire lives was to adjust one child and bring about that result in him—if that's all a chiropractor did in his or her entire life—I have absolutely no doubt that the chiropractor would say, "It's been worth becoming a chiropractor!"

David Singer, DC
David Singer Enterprises
Clearwater, Florida

Watch the Miracles

"There is always one moment in childhood when
the door opens and lets the future in."

Deepak Chopra

I'll never forget Brian. I first met the little charmer when he was two-years old, and I was in my first year of practice. Brian's diagnosis was cerebral palsy, and his parents had heard of me through my sister—then, as now, one of my biggest fans. As many do, they sought out Chiropractic care as a last resort.

Brian's prognosis was not good. At two, he had not yet sat up unsupported, much less stood. Although he had warm, loving, brown eyes that seemed to see and understand everything—as well as an infectious grin, he had poor or no motor control in his arms and legs. The source of Brian's condition was never really determined. Was it a birth defect? Had he suffered a lack of oxygen during the birth process? Was his problem due to excessive force used during delivery, resulting in injury? As is so often true in cases like this, there are more questions than answers. The frustration that develops from that state often paralyzes parents with fear. Fortunately, Brian's parents decided to try yet one more doctor: one with a different approach.

"Can you help our son?" It's such a simple question, really, yet so difficult to answer. The practical nature of the question is one thing; the emotional roller coaster—with its passengers of hopes, dreams, and fears—is something else. I did my best case history, consultation, and exam. I reviewed the records of the other doctors at the best hospitals and clinics. I looked up records of similar cases. And you know what? By the time I was done, I didn't know any more than the other doctors did. So my answer to his parents was this: "Our basic Chiropractic philosophy tells us that every person has a unique and substantial healing potential, and that the chief block to this potential is interference to the nervous system—the body's *controlling* system. I do find evidence of vertebral subluxation in your son, and relieving it with the gentlest of adjustments can help to release whatever his potential might be. The first law of healing is 'Do no harm,' and I know that what I do will either help or have no effect."

That day, I gave Brian his first Chiropractic adjustment. We made a game of it—as we do with all kids—and he was thrilled. He left as he came in, smiling in his mother's arms.

I had no sooner arrived in my office the next morning when Brian's parents called. They could hardly slow down enough to tell me the news. After Brian's adjustment the previous evening, they had gone home, had a little something to eat, and put the child to bed. Then they went into the living room to spend a few quiet moments together. Within minutes, they were startled by Brian's yells. They rushed into the nursery to find him standing in his crib, proudly holding onto the railing, and yelling at the top of his lungs! Needless to say, parents and child were ecstatic. But this was not the end of Brian's evening. After celebrating, crying, laughing, and thanking God, they put him back to sleep. Or so they thought. Brian proceeded to pull himself up in his crib over and over again that night, just as proud and happy as he could be.

From that moment on, Brian made rapid progress: sitting unsupported, being fitted for leg braces and learning to walk, talking, and developing his motor skills. With extra therapy and help, he went on to attend regular public school.

In a sense, we are all "Special Needs Children." We all have untapped potential inside. The nervous system not only controls every function of the body, it governs our perceptions as well. When it is free and clear of interference, we feel better, function better, learn better, and see the world in an entirely different light. Over the years, I've given more than 100,000 Chiropractic adjustments, and I've seen many, many lives change as a result.

Medical doctors, as a rule, do the best they can; but the art of prognosis is a tricky one. Here's what I've learned: never put limits on anyone's recovery...just remove the blocks, give nature a little nudge, then stand back and watch the miracles.

Peter W. Kfoury, DC, DABCI
Charleston, South Carolina

The Asthmatic Weatherman

Kelcey, a charming little boy who suffered from severe asthma, was six-years old when I first saw him. In the early 1990s, his family had been caught in a civil war marred by genocide in the African country of Burundi. The good news is that Kelcey's parents previously had been students at the California Polytechnic State University in San Luis Obispo (CalPoly for short) on California's Central Coast. Since the boy and his sister had been born in the United States while their parents were CalPoly students, that made the children U.S. citizens! Later, when the civil war in Burundi broke out, the U.S. government evacuated the entire family and they returned to San Luis Obispo.

Unfortunately, while the U.S. government had it together enough to get the family out (thereby saving their lives—a very nice benefit of U.S. citizenship), the government didn't have it together enough to issue green cards to the parents so that they could work and support themselves! Because Kelcey's parents weren't citizens and had no legal documents (emergency wartime evacuations rarely allow time for such formalities), they couldn't qualify for government aid. Essentially, the entire family was living off the generosity of people in their church.

My patient, Jean, mentioned Kelcey one day and lamented that it was too bad he couldn't get Chiropractic care to help his asthma. I asked how the family paid for medical doctors and was told that those doctors donated their services to the family. I realized in that moment that there are times when it is appropriate to donate services and told Jean I would be honored to see if I could help.

Soon thereafter, Kelcey came into the office, had an exam, and started under my care. While taking his history, I found out he'd been in the hospital several times each year due to acute asthma attacks. These attacks always seemed to be triggered by changes in the weather—especially the climate effects associated with impending rain. After a couple of weeks, Kelcey's mom noticed an improvement in his breathing and began backing off his asthma medication. He was progressing nicely and responding as expected.

On an early August afternoon, Kelcey and his mom came into the office for his usual adjustment. The weather was slightly muggy since we had had a freak rainstorm that morning—very unusual for that time of year in our area. When I asked Kelcey's mother how he was doing, she began to cry. Through tears and smiles she told me, "Ever since Kelcey has been alive, he has had severe asthma attacks just before it rains. Today is the first day of his life that I didn't know it was going to rain!" We all hugged and cried together.

Leslie Kasanoff, DC
Family Chiropractic and Wellness Center
Los Osos, California

7

Recovering
Sight and Hearing

"The child with his sweet pranks, the fool of his senses, commanded by every *sight* and *sound*, without any power to compare and rank his sensations, abandoned to a whistle or a painted chip, to a lead dragoon, or a gingerbread dog, individualizing everything, generalizing nothing, delighted with every new thing, lies down at night overpowered by the fatigue, which this day of continual pretty madness has incurred. But Nature has answered her purpose with the curly, dimpled lunatic. She has tasked every faculty, and has secured the symmetrical growth of the bodily frame, by all these attitudes and exertions—an end of the first importance, which could not be trusted to any care less perfect than her own."

Ralph Waldo Emerson
(1803-1882)

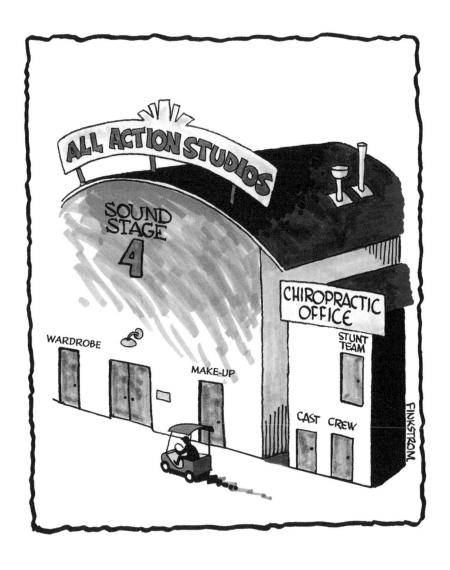

Reprinted by arrangement with Finkstrom Licensing International

Blind at Birth

"I once was lost, but now I'm found; was blind, but now I see." This well-known refrain from "Amazing Grace" speaks volumes about the incredible gift of God's grace toward *all* of mankind. Yet, speaking for myself, this timeless hymn not only carries with it hope for guidance and assurance from God above; it also contains a meaning that is nothing short of literal. I know, because I was blind at birth!

Initially, my condition was overlooked by the staff of the hospital where I was born. After all, obstetricians aren't trained to look for problems with their patient's sensory perceptions; they focus on *overall* indicators of health. Nevertheless, within the first few days of my life, Mom's maternal instincts told her something was wrong. While attending to routine care such as cuddling, feeding, and changing diapers, she found it unsettling that I never tried to make eye contact. After an extensive and frustrating search for an ophthalmologist who would even *look* at my case, my parents were presented with devastating news: their newborn daughter was completely blind due to improper neurological development.

In spite of this dismal prognosis, a small miracle took place after I entered my toddler years. Slowly-but-surely, I began to develop limited vision. I remember "seeing" just well enough to move about and play without outside assistance—and without bumping into things. I recall looking through one of my mother's books as a preschooler. From my young perspective, each white page was uniformly splattered with small-but-identical black dots. I remember thinking that "grown-ups" must really be smart in order to make sense out of this weird code.

When I was finally old enough to start school, my troubles *really* began. Teachers and classmates were often frustrated by my inability to function like fully-sighted children. My parents did the best they could to help and took me to every specialist they could find. Sadly, the answer was always the same: "Your daughter is legally blind with a visual acuity of 20/200. There is no treatment, cure, *or hope* for her condition."

And so it went throughout my childhood and adolescence. I simply had to muddle through social and academic pursuits without the benefit of full vision. From my perspective, matters became infinitely worse when tenth-grade rolled around: many of my peers got their driver's licenses. My inability to complete this rite-of-passage and enjoy the freedom and autonomy it conferred caused me to slip into depression. In fact, my despair led to severe, painful, and debilitating stomach ulcers. Once again, my parents took me to the best specialist they could find. The gastroenterologist pronounced my condition "incurable." What's more, even though I was only sixteen, he predicted I'd need to take prescription ulcer drugs for the rest of my life.

Once I graduated from high school and started attending college, I knew I needed part-time employment. Since I couldn't drive, I had to find a job within easy walking distance from home. An acquaintance worked at a chiropractor's office down the road and told me they needed a part-time receptionist for a new chiropractor on the staff. I remember thinking to myself, "*Chiropractors? Aren't they those weird doctors that move people's bones around?*" Even though I didn't have much knowledge about this type of practice—nor did I necessarily have a positive impression about their methods of patient care—I *did* need a job; this would have to do!

On my first day of work, I met the new—quite handsome, I might add—chiropractor whose receptionist I would become. He explained that one of my job requirements would be to make myself familiar with Chiropractic from a patient's perspective. That included being adjusted on a regular basis.

Honestly, I was scared. I already had more than enough physical problems; the last thing I needed was for someone to mess me up worse than I already was. To my pleasant surprise, not only did my neck and back suddenly begin to feel better; my "incurable" ulcers mysteriously disappeared. Of course, I immediately stopped taking the ulcer medication, thus—as an added bonus—freeing my body from the drug's unpleasant, inevitable, side effects!

Over the next couple of years, I continued working. I also received regular spinal adjustments. Strangely enough, I began to notice that my vision was improving. This made me wonder if I was starting to lose my mind. Maybe, since some other things were improving in my life, I was just imagining it. Years earlier, a chorus of leading specialists from the very best hospitals imperiously proclaimed: "Young lady, your vision will *never* improve!" But, since it never hurts to have a vision checkup, I scheduled one. Much to everyone's shock, the impossible had occurred. For the first time in twenty years, my vision had improved to 20/100, thus upgrading my diagnosis from "legally blind" to "visually-impaired." Smile, if you must, but this *little change* was a BIG DEAL for me!

Needless to say, I made regularly-scheduled adjustments a high priority from that point on. Over the next five years, my vision improved to 20/70. Thanks to Chiropractic, I now lead a normal, healthy, and productive life—including being able to drive! How did I thank that handsome chiropractor for the miracle he brought into my life? *I married him!* Now, twenty years and four vibrantly-healthy children later, we still work together in his office bringing Chiropractic miracles to the lives of others.

Laura S. Hattier
Proud wife and patient of
Donald G. Hattier, DC
Beachview Chiropractic Center
Millville, Delaware

Legible Handwriting and a Whole Lot More

"The highlight of my childhood was making my brother laugh so hard that food came out of his nose."

Gary Edward "Garrison" Keillor
Author, Storyteller, Humorist, and
Host of the Minnesota Public Radio program
A Prairie Home Companion®

Stephen appeared to be a healthy baby, just like our first two children. As Stephen got older, though, my husband and I noticed that he was having difficulty focusing on objects. We also noticed that something was different with Stephen when compared to our other two children. We took him in for an evaluation and were informed that he had *esatropia* and *strabismus*. These conditions prevent the muscles of the eyes from working correctly and thus affect visual function. Subsequently, Stephen had eye surgery and was fitted with bifocal eyeglasses, which he still wears to this day.

Although Stephen had eye complications, he continued to develop normally, just like any child his age. At two-years of age, Stephen had another stroke of bad luck. While at daycare one afternoon, a stray dog ferociously attacked him. The dog fractured Stephen's skull. Our son had to have another surgery to repair the damage. After the accident, Stephen healed well;

and my husband and I felt he would be on the road to normal childhood development.

Stephen began kindergarten at age five. Once he began school, my husband and I quickly realized there was something wrong with his learning abilities. Academically, Stephen wasn't learning quite as well as his brother and sister did at the same age. We hoped this would only be temporary, and, with a little help, he would catch up with the rest of his class.

When Stephen began first grade, he was tested and labeled, "learning disabled." Stephen had what they called a "perceptual communicative disorder." Although his IQ was tested at an "above average" level, he couldn't perform simple reading and writing tasks for his teachers. He had fine motor neurological deficits, and, because of this, reading and writing were his weaknesses. Stephen's handwriting was simply illegible and well below the skill level normal for his age. He began a special education program for his reading and written language. He was also seen by an occupational therapist for his fine motor complications.

As Stephen matured, we saw improvements in his reading and ability to get thoughts down on paper. However, much of his handwriting was still too difficult to read, and, to us as parents, still of concern. When Stephen was halfway through fifth grade, we had not given up trying to help our son overcome his reading and writing obstacles. With middle school only a year-and-a-half away, we were still looking for something or someone to help make a difference in our child's life.

I had heard about Chiropractic healthcare helping children in many ways. Friends and acquaintances had mentioned Chiropractic helping kids with headaches, ear infections, and even ADD. I wasn't really sure if Chiropractic care could help our son. Neither my husband nor I had ever been to a chiropractor before, and we had limited first-hand knowledge about it. I contacted Dr. Trevor Van Wyk, a local chiropractor, to see if there was any scientific research showing that Chiropractic care improved fine motor problems. He assured me that there was; and we decided to have Dr. Van Wyk take care of Stephen.

Dr. Van Wyk did a Chiropractic evaluation and informed us that our child had a condition in his spine called subluxation. The doctor informed us that Stephen had subluxations in several areas of his spine. He told us that the first bone in Stephen's neck was severely misaligned and rotated, and that this was interfering with his nerve function. Dr. Van Wyk told us that he could make the subluxation areas of our child's spine improve by delivering Chiropractic adjustments. This would restore nerve function, thus bringing about the possibility of an improvement in Stephen's fine motor skills. He felt that if the fine motor problems improved, Stephen's handwriting would also improve. Dr. Van Wyk gave us no guarantees, but with nothing to lose, we told him to start adjusting our son.

As of this writing, Stephen has been under Dr. Van Wyk's care for about three months. We have already seen wonderful improvements in several areas of Stephen's life. For one, he has become a much calmer child. It has always been difficult for Stephen to sit still during dinner or while doing his homework. Since he started receiving Chiropractic adjustments, Stephen is able to sit still and be more relaxed. We've also noticed that Stephen is able to concentrate much better while doing tasks and homework. He also used to stay up until late hours of the evening until his teenage brother and sister went to bed—often-times after 10:00pm. He now sleeps more soundly; is not as restless; and—to *everyone's* relief—snores much less. Finally, Stephen's handwriting has improved since he started Chiropractic care. We can now definitely read his very legible handwriting, and his calmer personality allows him to take the time to make sure it is legible.

Stephen still has a long way to go academically, but we do believe that Chiropractic care is helping our son make progress. In fact, all of our children and my husband and I are now receiving

Chiropractic care from Dr. Van Wyk, and we have all seen a big change in one or more areas of our lives. It is truly unfortunate that more people don't know about the benefits of Chiropractic health care. I know it has made a huge difference in the health of my family; why not let it make a difference in the health of yours?

Carolyn Paletta
Chiropractic advocate and
Mother of Stephen Paletta
A happy patient of
Trevor Van Wyk, DC
Van Wyk Family Chiropractic
Littleton, Colorado

A Life-Changing Event!

Eric Zack, our son, first met Dr. David Spear at the Lane County Fair in Oregon during which the doctor offered complimentary Chiropractic evaluations. Dr. David looked at my other child and found nothing to speak of. However, when he looked at Eric's posture, neck, back, etc., he began to ask me questions.

I'd never considered that something that happened at birth could have affected my eight-year-old, but it had. I scheduled a follow-up evaluation in the doctor's office and filled out the questionnaire on Eric's health that was mailed to me. The form read like Eric's medical record checklist: *Assisted birth—YES; chronic ear infections—YES; asthma—YES; allergies—YES; cavities—YES; glasses—YES; trouble sleeping—YES; trouble reading—YES.*

The list of my son's illnesses went on and on, and included six trips to the emergency room, two hospitalizations, a breathing machine at home, tutoring, and glasses. To minimize sources of allergens, we had moved, bought goats, and changed the entire family's diet. And we had spent many sleepless nights with a sick child. I cannot convey to you how many bizarre illnesses he's had. A partial list includes: blood-borne bacterial infection, "teenage mononucleosis"—*at four-years old,* fevers high enough to cause hallucinations, tubes in his ears, and rotted teeth due to the large amount of antibiotics he took. At seven, he was tested for rheumatoid arthritis due to his medical history and the bone spurs that had mysteriously appeared on his heels. All the while, my husband and I wondered, "What else can we do to help our son?"

We had sort of resigned ourselves to the view that Eric was "delicate" and "sensitive." As he got older and began school, the disappointment for us as parents continued. No matter that we volunteered in the classroom, read to him daily, and did everything recommend to "give your child a head start," the results were still disappointing. I was told he needed tutoring. He was at "high risk," but fell through the cracks to get help at school. He missed tons of classes, couldn't complete assignments on time, and got frustrated to the point of hating himself. It was awful. So we did hours and hours of $30 per session tutoring. Not even *that* was enough.

We took Eric to the optometrist hoping for someone to explain why life was so hard for the boy. We got a simple answer: he needed glasses! He had some sort of visual tracking issue that made it difficult for him to focus on anything—especially close up. Being optimistic parents, we were thrilled! But it didn't help as much as we had hoped. Eric felt awkward with the glasses on and would forget them. Of course, this just made him more irritated and frustrated. I took the summer off from my job. For his entire vacation, I didn't make Eric pick up a single book on his own. Of course, he was quite happy with that arrangement.

Around the end of August, I decided that if Eric could get by as a marginal student, he had enough great things going for him and that maybe he'd be okay. Although disappointed, I resigned myself to that prospect.

Then came the Lane County Fair and Dr. David. For the Zack family, that was *a life-changing event!* Dr. David met with each of us and took an exhaustive health history of Eric. Eric began Chiropractic care and initially saw the doctor three times a week for adjustments. Subsequently, his visit frequency gradually decreased due to Eric's steady improvement. Oh yeah, now for the *really good part!*

We noticed a change in Eric within the first two weeks. He played soccer better, got out of bed in the morning without the usual fuss, and was obviously a much happier boy. My husband and I discussed the improvement and decided to continue with Chiropractic because it seemed to be helping. Now came a big test: Flu Season! We got through it without a hitch. My daughter, who *never* gets sick, got the croup, but not Eric! We were amazed. His classmates were dropping like flies; he *did* not and *has* not missed one minute of school so far this year due to illness. His school health exam results came: eyes—perfect, ears—perfect! What? This was too weird—*impossible* even. So, back to the eye doctor we went to confirm this miracle of Chiropractic care.

Everyone in our family has seen the same eye doctor for the past two years, so he knows us pretty well. Likewise, we know him; he's skeptical, analytical, and very thorough. I entered the exam room with Eric and didn't let on that anything had changed. After about five minutes of examining him, Dr. Cleveland literally scratched his head and said, "If Eric were seeing me for the first time today, I would not prescribe glasses for him."

I began to tell the eye doctor about our work with Dr. David and how we had just stopped tutoring for Eric due to his dramatic improvement in reading. Dr. Cleveland told me that given the changes in Eric's eyes, he would expect his reading to improve dramatically in the coming months. He told me that he had never seen such a remarkable improvement in the eyes of a child this age! I was shocked—*but only for about two seconds*—based on the whole life turnaround Eric has had. I connected the two doctors, and they are talking about referrals and producing more clinical data like they saw in Eric—totally empirical data that shows this treatment works. I was sold! So the next week, it was time for yet another test: School Conferences.

Eric's teacher and I met; and she was thrilled. "Eric has improved so much since last spring it's amazing! Look at this!" She proceeded to show me example after example of his miraculous improvement in such a short time. But at this point, I expected this! Yippee! This is OUR story, *it is real* and *it is amazing.*

If you are the mother of a youngster, and if you had an assisted birth employing forceps, vacuum/suction, or some other "artificial" procedure—get your child checked by a chiropractor. Don't wait until they have lived the life Eric had to endure for eight years. The problems caused by assisted birth can be corrected when your children are young. Now that we've been through this ordeal, I'd like to shout it from the rooftops, fund a study, and do anything I can to help get the word out! If this is your family, your children, someone you know—*do something!* I'm happy to personally talk to anyone about Eric's transformation. The moral of the story is HUGE! I wonder how many children out there are in Eric's boat or worse: overmedicated, ill, discouraged, and uncoordinated. Get educated on the subject of children and Chiropractic care and change a life for the better.

Adapted from an article in
Pathways to Family Wellness magazine
by Christine B. Zack, CLTC
Mother of Eric Zack
A happy patient of
David Spear, PhD, DC and Melody Spear, DC
Body of Light Family Chiropractic
Eugene, Oregon

Amazing Side Effect

*Hope is the thing with feathers
That perches in the soul.
And sings the tune
Without the words,
and never stops at all.*

Emily Elizabeth Dickinson
American Poet
(1830-1886)

When asked if Chiropractic is "just for headaches and back-aches," many uninformed people would probably tell you "yes." But, for Karla, she gladly tells everyone who will listen that it's a *life-saving* way of life.

I first knew Karla's parents, Cheryl and Thomas, as my patients. Thomas was in a wheelchair when we met and couldn't feel from the waist down. After twelve years of Veterans Administration hospital care, he was still getting worse. Within three weeks of starting *Chiropractic* care, he was driving a car! His now-unneeded wheelchair is proudly on display in my clinic.

Cheryl was terribly worried about her daughter who had a whole list of serious health conditions. After seeing the amazing results her husband was getting, Cheryl wanted her daughter to start care as well. Karla, however, was afraid of Chiropractic and didn't want to participate. Cheryl was certain that Chiropractic was safe and would help her daughter, and she knew the only way to get her daughter into a chiropractor's clinic was to trick her.

Karla was well aware that her parents were my patients. One hot July day, Cheryl and Thomas had Karla come along to their regular maintenance adjustment appointments. Cheryl told Karla it was too hot to stay in the car and that she should come inside and wait until they were through. Her idea was that if I could just talk with Karla and answer some of her questions, she wouldn't be afraid any more. I was able to explain to a very skeptical young woman about the brain/nervous system that controls the whole body. That wherever there were subluxations—pinched nerves— there would also be a loss in communication and function between the brain and those affected body parts. I explained that my job as a chiropractor was to detect and correct subluxation for the health of the whole body and all its functions.

Karla agreed to an examination. When she began treatment, Karla was legally blind, suffered from persistent nausea, and had endured constant headaches for almost seven months. Lastly, her diabetes was out-of-control and slowly killing her. Her blood sugar monitor routinely registered "high"—which meant it was above the top-listed reading of six-hundred. She was on two different medications for headaches and was taking Reglan for nausea—a medicine given to chemotherapy patients. Karla had sustained kidney damage due to diabetes and was only filtering at fifty percent. She was told that more than eleven-hundred micro-units of protein were spilling over into her urine every day—a normal quantity is under two hundred.

I guess you could say the last condition Karla came in with was a spirit of hopelessness. She had been to, and through, all the con-ventional means of healthcare and was obviously dying. I asked if she expected to improve, stay the same, or get worse, if she contin-ued her then-current medical regimen. She admitted she realized she was getting worse. I then asked if she would give Chiropractic a try since it was non-invasive, required no drugs, and produced only one side-effect: *improved health!* As a last resort, she agreed.

Three weeks after Karla started regular Chiropractic adjustments, she was completely off her headache medicine. After two more weeks, she was off the Reglan. I'd have her take a blood sugar reading before her adjustment and traction and then again immediately afterward. Routinely, it would drop 50 to 60 points. Now, when she takes a reading before her adjustment, it never registers over 300, and the numbers are still improving. Her kidney function has, so far, improved to 60% with her protein levels still dropping. Additionally, the last time she went to have her eyes checked, her vision was blurring because her glass prescription had become too strong for her improving eyesight. Her ophthalmologist has documented the improvement.

All these health changes are, of course, wonderful; but seeing the look of purpose, hope, and life in Karla's face is the icing on the cake.

Bill E. Hannouche, DC
Hannouche Family Chiropractic Clinic
Spartanburg, South Carolina

I Can See Clearly Now!

"All my life through, the new sights of Nature made me rejoice like a child."

Madame Marie Curie
Two-time Nobel Laureate: Physics and Chemistry
(1867-1934)

For several years, I suffered with daily headaches. At least twice per month, usually during stressful situations, my headaches were so severe that I had sharp pains behind and around my right eye. The right side of my neck was painful, as were my shoulder muscles and the area between my shoulder blades. In addition to these problems, I was plagued with fatigue and occasional radiating pain down my right leg. I was a member of a singing quartet and a trio, and my symptoms were making it extremely difficult for me to pursue my favorite hobbies.

A friend of mine, who had been diagnosed with fibromyalgia and had found relief through Chiropractic care, suggested that I consult her doctor. I met with Dr. Clifford Hardick, and his x-rays of my spine identified severe subluxations in my lower back and an unusual curvature in my neck. Dr. Hardick explained that while a healthy neck has a forward curvature, mine was reversed. This condition contributed to my headaches, shoulder pain, and neck pain. It was obvious from the x-rays that my spinal problems could not be corrected overnight.

Two weeks after beginning Chiropractic care, the frequency of my headaches started to diminish. I felt much better. However, one month into care, I began to notice that the vision in my left eye was becoming blurry. As a matter of fact, my vision was blurriest immediately following an adjustment. The problem continued for a number of weeks. After a Chiropractic adjustment, I would return to work and have dizzy spells because of the blurred vision. In spite of these unusual circumstances, and in spite of others' suggestions that Chiropractic care was possibly causing a new problem for me, Dr. Hardick knew well that my subluxations were being reduced; so he continued to adjust me.

On Dr. Hardick's recommendation, I visited an optometrist who found that I had a dilated pupil in my left eye. At the time, vascular disorders, diabetes, and multiple sclerosis were all explained to me as possible causes. Another specialist suggested that the enlarged pupil was harmless, and that it may have been caused by a virus. And yet another specialist suggested that my blurred vision was being caused by an Adie's eye, an eye with a pupil that reacts very sluggishly to light.

After six months of Chiropractic care, my headaches were extremely rare, and the occasional symptom was always alleviated immediately following an adjustment. At this time, Dr. Hardick's new x-ray of my neck showed a normal, healthy, forward curve in my neck. The major goal of my Chiropractic care had been achieved.

However, my vision was still blurry. In fact, it was actually getting *blurrier!* Dr. Hardick insisted that I see an optometrist to have my vision measured. I went to the optometrist's office wearing a strong pair of -8 eyeglasses for nearsightedness, the glasses I had been wearing prior to my first Chiropractic appointment. I left the optometrist's office with a new prescription: -4. Yes, my vision had *improved* with Chiropractic care! It was my overpowered lenses that were blurring my vision. After months of appointments with optometrists, neurologists, and ophthalmologists, I finally had my answer.

Improved eyesight was the last thing I expected to receive as a "side effect" of Chiropractic care. With regular adjustments, I have the health and energy to work full time, sing every weekend, and enjoy my everyday activities.

My optometrist now asks me to get adjusted immediately before having my vision tested. I recommend that you do the same.

Sheila Jackson
Chiropractic advocate
Grateful patient of
B. J. Hardick, DC
Hardick Chiropractic Centre
London, Ontario
CANADA

Dr. Hardick is the co-author of
Maximized Living Nutrition Plans

Can You Hear Me Now?

I walked into my treatment room one morning and observed a well-dressed, elderly lady I'd never seen before. Seated, she was bent over, busily filling out a new patient form attached to a clipboard in her lap. "Hello!" I said. No response. "Hello!" I said again—in a much louder voice. She turned, slowly raised her head, and looked at me with a faint smile. I quickly noticed two large, unattractive hearing aids, one protruding from each ear.

After I shook her hand and introduced myself, I began my standard new patient interview. Her form identified the lady as Agnes, age 78. I carefully studied her health history and saw that her chief complaint was general neck pain and stiffness. Agnes explained that the onset of her pain had been gradual over the previous several years, that it was not due to any particular trauma or injury she could remember, and that she had tried physical therapy and medication for relief—to no avail. I had to nearly shout my questions because of her hearing impairment.

I next performed an examination and x-ray, noting her restricted range of neck movement, knotted muscles in spasm, fixation of joint movement, and arthritic degeneration of the discs in her neck. After a thorough review of my findings, I recommended that we begin adjusting Agnes. She agreed. I then carefully positioned her on my treatment table and performed an adjustment to her seventh cervical vertebra. When I later bid her goodbye, I shouted, *"Come back in two days for a followup visit!"*

As instructed, Agnes dutifully returned two days later. When I entered the treatment room, the first thing I noticed was that she was standing with her right arm extended. At the end of her arm was a menacing, clenched fist—knuckles up and pointed in my direction! For a moment, she scared me!

Soon after, I realized my fear was completely unjustified. Tears were streaming down Agnes' face. My melancholic nature immediately made me wonder if I'd done something to make her suffer.

Agnes slowly opened her hand, palm-up, and revealed two hearing aids—the same ugly ear adornments I had noticed on her first visit. "Doctor," she said, "ever since you adjusted my neck just two days ago, *I don't need these anymore!*"

I was awestruck! I'd learned in my Chiropractic training that the profession began in 1895 when a Dr. Daniel Palmer adjusted the neck of a man named Harvey Lillard, alleviating his deafness. More than a hundred years later, I had replicated Palmer's adjustment with a similar result!

Agnes went on to explain that her hearing had slowly diminished over a period of several years, and that she had recently purchased the most powerful hearing aids available. She gleefully continued by saying that soon after my adjustment, she began noticing her hearing aids were too loud and bothersome. When she removed them, she discovered she had near-perfect hearing.

Restraining as much of my excitement as I could, I explained that there are delicate "trophic" nerves that exit the spine in the area I had adjusted. These nerves join the main auditory nerve that facilitates hearing. I continued, "Those trophic nerves were probably pinched—contributing to your hearing problem. The adjustments simply removed pressure on the nerves."

Agnes hugged me and thanked me as we both wept with joy. Then, we both laughed when she said her neck had definitely *not* improved. Mightily impressed with the progress she experienced after just one adjustment, however, she continued her "hearing treatment" over several weeks and, in the process, obtained significant relief for her neck pain as well.

Appreciating that periodic Chiropractic adjustments can help maintain health, Agnes decided to continue receiving care from me on a monthly basis. She remained my patient for another twelve years. On each and every visit, whenever I adjusted Agnes, I always checked her ears. Those hearing aids were never seen again.

Tom Potisk, DC
aka The "Down-to-Earth" Doctor
www.thedowntoearthdoctor.com
Caledonia, Wisconsin

8

Patient Comeback Stories

"It is most necessary to know the nature of the spine.
One or more vertebrae may or may not go out of
place very much and if they do, they are likely
to produce serious complications and even
death, if not properly adjusted. Many
diseases are related to the spine."

Hippocrates
Greek Father of Medicine
after whom the Hippocratic Oath is named
(460-357 BC)

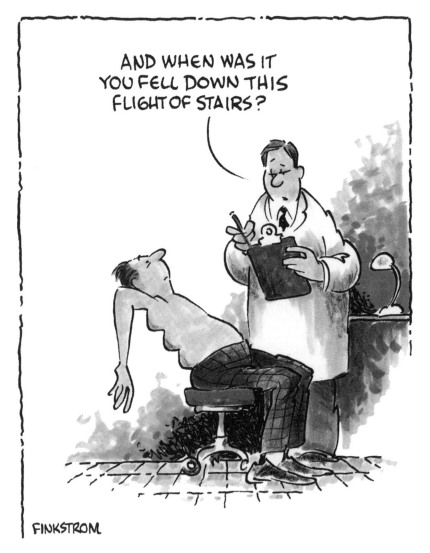

Reprinted by arrangement with Finkstrom Licensing International

I Just Want to Walk Again!

One afternoon in 1988, a desperate young woman called from New York City to my high rise Chiropractic practice in Houston. Our receptionist immediately transferred the call to my back consultation office where I was reviewing patient films.

In a tear-filled voice, the caller said, "Dr. Demartini, you don't know who I am, but Carlos, my boyfriend, and his mother are patients of yours."

"Is Carlos the aspiring young actor?" I asked.

"Yes."

"What's happened? You sound frantic and scared!"

"Carlos has been in a serious car accident. The doctors don't know if he's going to live. He severed his cervical spinal cord, and he can't move. He's completely paralyzed."

"Okay, what would you love for me to do? How can I be of help? Do you want me to fly up to meet with him? What are you requesting?"

"Doctor, I don't exactly know *what* I'm asking. All I know is that his mother begged me to call you."

I tried to calm the distraught woman: "Please gather all of Carlos's medical records into a folder and send the collection to me so I can study his case, find out what's happened, what is being done, what is *going* to be done, and whether it would be helpful for me to fly to Manhattan—something I'd gladly do if I thought I could help."

With a sigh of relief, she said, "Okay, I'll do that."

I assumed she would call back relatively soon. But I did *not* hear back from her right away. In fact, I don't know *what* transpired afterwards, and—in those pre-cell phone days—I had no way to contact her.

A full six months later, this same lady phoned again: "Dr. Demartini, the New York hospital is transporting Carlos to a hospital in Houston. Eventually, he'll move in with his mom for special care."

I told her, "Just let me know when you get here, and I'll visit Carlos."

When Carlos was finally relocated to his mother's home, the lady called again. This time, she scheduled an appointment to bring Carlos in to see me. When they arrived at my front reception desk, Carlos was strapped very carefully into a special quadriplegic wheelchair. His head was harnessed, and his body was paralyzed from the neck down. When they wheeled him into my consultation office, Carlos was lightly medicated and very solemn. His eyes were cast down and the lady told me he was feeling hopeless, depressed, and—yes—*suicidal*. Carlos's inner dream had been to become a great actor, to dance, and to perform in theater and movies. He wanted to act on Broadway and dance in musicals. But there he was—in a *quadriplegic wheelchair!*

I looked at him and said, "Carlos! What are you thinking and feeling *inside? Talk* to me!"

"*I just want to* walk *again!*" he replied. "I just want to *dance* again. I just want to *act* again. I don't want to live any longer if I have to remain like *this!*"

I looked at the young man, let him continue speaking, and encouraged him to vent his frustration.

Then I said, "Carlos, if you have a determined *will* to live, if you have a strong *desire* to return to greater function, and if you *believe* in the possibility of having some kind of recovery, then—and only then—will you have the necessary elements with which to achieve success. *And I will help you get there!* It's essential that you have some meaningful and inspiring vision to work toward.

You'll require a clear, qualitative dream to activate your nervous system toward such an empowering objective. Because if you *don't* have a will to live, and only have a will to *die*, then you're *already* defeated! Do you truly have the will necessary to overcome your potential challenges and obstacles? I need to have your complete commitment if I'm going to work with you and—together—we'll achieve something extraordinary with your mind and body. Whatever results we create out of working together, whatever we can improve, I want to make sure that you have something driving you to succeed far beyond the ordinary."

Carlos made his decision immediately and with enthusiasm: "*Yes, Doctor, I want to do it!* I just want to walk again, dance again, and act again."

"Well, then," I said, "let's go! Let's begin your life-changing, body-empowering Chiropractic care."

First, I examined Carlos's spine, reviewed his large stack of radiographs, read his mountain of previous test results, and formulated a treatment plan for his remarkable recovery. Next, I began to carefully and gently adjust certain portions of his cervical (upper) spine. At first, I didn't want to adjust him too forcibly because his neck had wires and bolts all through it. One afternoon, after working with Carlos almost every day for weeks and not achieving the results that I initially had hoped for, I laid him on my adjusting table and informed him that, "I'm going to more forcibly adjust this one primary vertebra that is completely restricted and subluxated and that has been firmly wired in a position slightly out of alignment."

Of course, I was a bit anxious because, in my rational mind, adjusting this wired-and-restricted vertebra seemed partially *irrational* and possibly *contraindicated*. But something intuitive whispered to me, "Adjust *this* one; this one is *the key!*"

Well, I adjusted this single cervical vertebra that had been fractured and displaced the most. On the night following this adjustment, Carlos began to feel his toes for the first time since the accident. The next day, I adjusted him again, and he was able to partially control his own bladder. I adjusted him almost every day and—over the next six months—not only was he able to begin moving his toes, feet, and legs, and regain some control over his bowel; he was starting to move his hands and upper torso. His newly-enabled upper-torso movement enhanced his ability to breathe independently. In fact, Carlos's adjustments were changing his entire physiology.

Then, after about nine months of steady Chiropractic care, Carlos experienced a major psychological breakthrough. I had just completed his latest adjustment and was about to leave for Dallas to speak at a Chiropractic Research Seminar. As I was exiting the adjusting room, Carlos called out: "Dr. Demartini, I have a surprise for you. I'm going to *walk* when you return next week!"

At that moment, I was a bit taken aback and didn't quite know how to respond. Part of me was thinking, "*That's* a bit of a stretch," and yet I couldn't say anything but "*Great!* That's the spirit and the determination of a *champion!*"

At the three-day weekend conference, I eagerly shared with my Chiropractic colleagues the results-to-date of my experience with Carlos. After my return to Houston, I found myself once again treating this remarkable, willpower-driven patient. After receiving his focused adjustment, and true to his word of the previous week, Carlos eased himself off the table—unassisted, and—with the help of gravity—swung into his wheelchair. Then—with no assistance but the use of his own hands and arms, he carefully leaned forward and grabbed the edge of the countertop. Very slowly, he "walked" his bottom to the front edge of the wheelchair seat and began to pull himself up. With shaking legs, he gradually leaned forward until he was completely upright. Then, he turned toward me and attempted a few faltering steps. Within moments, he started a slow-motion fall into my waiting arms. These were the first steps Carlos had attempted since his near-fatal car crash! I can't adequately describe my emotions as I witnessed this heroic effort. But I wasn't the only one inspired by the scene; most of my staff developed "leaky eyeballs" as we watched.

Over the next few months, Carlos developed the ability to hobble, hunched over, with a cane. Sometimes, he would even tuck the cane under his arm, stand erect, and slowly *walk!* The original doctors said he would forever remain paralyzed. They said he would never move or have any normal function. But here he is, today, walking and functioning independently.

I don't believe that any doctor truly has the right to tell a patient, "There's no way you'll ever be able to do...again." No doctor truly knows the limits of an inspired human mind and body. All I know is that—because of his vision, determination, and Chiropractic adjustments—Carlos is walking once again.

Carlos never did fully recover his ability to act or dance. But—as a *teacher*—he has assisted a number of others in doing so. Today, it is through the lives of his students that Carlos is able to fulfill his performing arts dreams.

John F. Demartini, DC
Founder
The Demartini Institute

Dr. Demartini is the bestselling author of
*Count Your Blessings—
The Healing Power of Gratitude and Love*

Firefighter: Every Kid's Dream

> "Two and three years after patients with back pain were treated by chiropractors, they experienced far less pain than those who were treated by medical doctors."
>
> BMJ (British Medical Journal), 1990
> (an international peer reviewed medical journal)

Like any typical younger brother, I followed my big brother everywhere. One of the places I'd follow him to was the town Volunteer Fire Station. It wasn't long before I started attending training classes. At the age of sixteen, I started riding the big red trucks to fires with the sirens screeching and the emergency lights flashing—*every kid's dream!* For the next fourteen years, I dedicated all my spare time to protecting the people of our community.

By the early 80s, our town had grown so large that the taxpayers could afford a full-time fire department. Thirty-two-years of age at that point, in excellent physical shape, and having plenty of experience, I applied for a position. Soon after, I received an appointment as a firefighter with the rank of private. That was one of the happiest days of my life; and I looked forward to a long and fulfilling career!

Two years into my service, on a cold February day, I helped move a heavy patient into a rescue truck. When I lifted, I felt a shooting pain in my back. The next morning, I experienced excruciating pain in my left lower back, buttocks, and legs.

For the following nine months, I embarked on an ever-more-discouraging medical journey through the offices of numerous doctors and physical therapists. Diagnostic tests including MRI, Myelogram, CT scan, and EEG were administered. Medications prescribed included an assortment of pain killers, muscle relaxants, and anti-inflammatory drugs. I also received 21 separate injections (including cortisone) into my lower back. Nothing helped, and I was afraid that I'd have to take early retirement from the job I loved. My neurosurgeon said there was nothing more he could do. I was told to live with the pain and take pain killers when needed. Naturally, I refused to accept this prognosis, so the neurosurgeon suggested I consider Chiropractic! In fact, he was the man that referred me to Drs. Edward Caputo and Judith Gallagher.

I called Dr. Caputo's office on a Monday and had a consultation the next day. I made clear from the start that I was suffering from severe back and leg pain. The staff immediately made a favorable impression on me. They were friendly, professional, and eager to help. Following a thorough examination, Dr. Caputo determined that my pain was due to a lack of stability in my lower back. He became my primary doctor with Dr. Gallagher assisting. They said they were sure they could help me—*if* I was willing to help myself.

In a typical early session, I received Chiropractic adjustments administered by Dr. Caputo plus hot and cold therapy, electrical stimulation, back-stretching exercises, and another exercise that helped me immensely: walking in a pool. I learned that a one-mile walk in the water equals two and a half miles on land. My initial plan called for three visits a week, and—as I improved—was reduced to two times per week. All the adjustments were pain-free.

Approximately twelve weeks after the start of treatment, I returned to work. Forced early retirement was no longer a concern! Instead, I looked forward to taking the promotional exam for lieutenant. Six months after my first visit with Dr. Caputo, I was awarded that promotion. I continued to do well, with stretching and aqua therapy being the key along with periodic "maintenance" Chiropractic adjustments. Several years later, I was promoted to captain. Unquestionably, Drs. Caputo and Gallagher made my career as a firefighter possible. Their compassionate, knowledgeable care not only healed my back; it also healed my spirit.

David Dinobile
Grateful patient of
Edward Caputo, DC
and
Judith Gallagher, DC
Caputo Chiropractic
Cranston, Rhode Island

The Circle of Wellness: Rodney's Story

In 23 years of Chiropractic practice, I've been blessed to meet many extraordinary people and have worked on hundreds of interesting cases. One involved a patient—now a friend—named Rodney. A former heavyweight boxer and security officer, Rod is a *mountain* of a man standing six feet, seven inches tall in his stocking feet! While working a security detail one night, Rod was hit with seven lead slugs from a high-caliber weapon. Miraculously surviving the ambush, he had to endure multiple, delicate operations over the next two years as surgeons attempted to repair the damage.

Rod's experience exacted a *mental*—as well as a physical—toll. To treat his psychological trauma, Rod was directed to the care of a counselor who happened to be another patient of mine. In short order, the counselor referred Rod to me. The referral was made not only so we could treat Rod's persistent, excruciating back pain—two gunshot-caused herniated discs sustained during the ambush, but also so that Rod could benefit from our stress management course—part of the "Circle of Wellness" program we offer at Lavanga Chiropractic.

As with most of our new patients, Rod had never been to a chiropractor before, but he wasn't the type of person who had much trepidation about anything. His history revealed several issues that he wanted me to address: the herniated discs and associated back pain, a constant stiffness in his neck and shoulders, and throbbing headaches. He was taking serial courses of antibiotics due to unhealed wounds in his stomach that caused sudden diarrhea plus occasional incontinence and impotency. He was on daily blood pressure, cholesterol, and antidepressant medications, and had to cope with unrelenting mental tension and anger toward his attacker. In spite of all this, what I discovered in my first encounter was a truly authentic human being with a tremendous sense of self and an irrepressible sense of humor; Rod was a textbook "Gentle Giant"!

We began with a comprehensive evaluation to determine the current cause of his symptoms. While gunshots were the obvious *initial* cause, I explained to Rod that his body had already been through at least one healing cycle and would perhaps need to complete two—or even three—more. Only then would we know the full extent of his remaining issues and be able to formulate an accurate prognosis. I also discussed with Rod our center's philosophy and related it to our treatment recommendations and a follow-through plan for him.

I explained to Rod that since its inception in 1895, Chiropractic was meant to be more than a manipulation to align the spine and restore balance and health. It is a *lifestyle*, a way of thinking and living in tune with nature. I showed Rod the Circle of Wellness chart we use at our center that explains the seven facets of healing: Chiropractic, Massage, Exercise, Detoxification, Nutrition, Stress Management, and Coaching—the elements that define our mission and method of delivering Chiropractic care.

With Rod's agreement and participation, we laid out a strategy that would see him through his cycles of healing in an effective and non-invasive manner. We scheduled a series of adjustments and massages, encouraged him to resume the basic exercises that boxers perform, and added a few stretches from our Yoga instructor to restore his flexibility. Rod completed a detox program to rid his body of toxins and was persuaded to eliminate toxic food and drink from his diet in order to balance his systemic pH (acid and base levels).

Next, we formulated a basic nutritional program for Rod that included multi-vitamin, B-complex, D3, and Omega 3 supplements plus extra iron and calcium. We also added probiotics to counteract Rod's daily antibiotics regimen and CoQ10 to counterbalance the muscle pain brought on by the statin drugs he was taking to lower cholesterol. In addition, we went to work on his *thinking game*. I told Rod my hope was that someday he would step on stage with me at one of my seminars and tell his *story of gratitude* for the ambush that almost killed him but gave him a new way of looking at life and love. We taught him our stress management tool, The Demartini Method® —developed by Dr. John F. Demartini, to help Rod perfect his ability to deal with who he is as a person now and especially to overcome the understandable anger and hatred he felt for his attacker. It was a complete Chiropractic Circle of Wellness strategy.

Within a matter of *days*, Rod began to feel better physically. In weeks he started to enjoy little activities with his son that he had been unable to do previously. Within *six months*, his bowel situation was coming under control, and he no longer complained about the anxiety of having to always be near a bathroom. In *less than a year*, he was off blood pressure, cholesterol, and antidepressant medications. Approximately *eighteen months* after his first visit, Rod did the unthinkable: he returned to work. Although he was physically weaker, he was mentally stronger!

Now, four-plus years since I first met Rod, he is 90% recovered and healthy enough to exercise rigorously. Another indicator of his progress is that he's gotten married; I was privileged to be a guest at his wedding. Rod and his wife are now the proud parents of two healthy children, a boy and a girl.

Rod attributes much of his comeback to Chiropractic and me. While I agree about the Chiropractic aspect, I give the rest of the credit for his recovery to Rod and God.

Daniel F. Lavanga, DC
Lavanga Chiropractic
Feasterville, Pennsylvania

Margaret's Story

In 1995, when I started practicing Chiropractic in Australia, one of my first patients was a 33-year-old woman named Margaret. Asked to complete her medical history questionnaire, she ticked almost all of the boxes on the form and used the space in the margins to note additional complaints. We then moved to the next phase of her healing process, a same-visit interview during which we formally discussed her condition.

Margaret explained that her medical doctor had recently said her health was so bad she'd soon be on a pension and would have to give up work entirely. Her questionnaire revealed that while undergoing a simple surgical procedure (under anesthesia) at age 26, she had experienced *three* heart attacks and subsequently fell into a coma. When she revived, Margaret's physicians told her she had also suffered a stroke resulting in paroxysmal supra-ventricular tachycardia (PSVT: a permanent, spasmodic condition characterized by brief-but-uncomfortable episodes of very rapid heart rate). Another significant medical problem of which Margaret complained was right-arm numbness. This was the result of an improperly-placed intravenous needle that missed the intended blood vessel and permanently injured the nerves and associated musculature of her right arm.

A year after her botched surgery, Margaret slipped and fell on a wet floor at work. This resulted in back and hip injuries after which she was placed on workers compensation. Following this mishap, Margaret often used a cane to help her walk. However, even after three months off for recuperation, her condition did not improve. No malingerer, she insisted on returning to work; but her symptoms began to worsen.

Margaret and I continued to review her "brief" medical history form on which she stated that, after the fall, she started experiencing severe cramps in her low back. The cramps caused spasms so intense they'd make her scream and cry. The extreme discomfort produced poor sleep patterns as she could never get comfortable. The sciatic pain shot down her leg and, when attempting to walk, she couldn't put weight on her right foot to *stand*, much less *walk!* Margaret was always fatigued and anxious and regularly had to stop and rest. She was troubled by constant headaches, neck and jaw pain, dizzy spells, and stress. Often constipated, she also had challenges with Candida (yeast infections) due to the constant administration of antibiotics.

As our new-patient interview continued, Margaret explained that—in addition to the stroke and heart damage resulting from her simple surgery, she suffered from asthma, severe arthritis, bronchitis, chronic cystitis (bladder infections), skin rashes, and polycystic ovaries. She was on a *huge* number of drugs and was served by doctors in almost every specialty including cardiology, orthopedics, rheumatology, pulmonology, allergy, anesthetics, podiatry, gynecology, dermatology, and now, Chiropractic.

Margaret was miserable, and typically grumpy and abrupt in her manner. Fiercely independent, she often alienated her family and friends as a result of her pain-driven, aggressive manner. Her job was *really* important to her as it gave her a reason to get up each morning. To Margaret, the thought of not working was *terrifying!*

After my initial consultation with Margaret, I asked myself, "Where do I start," and, "What could I do?" I knew I needed to treat the *person*, not the *problem*. Throughout my diagnostic process, I was guided by what I had learned in college: "The *gem* of Chiropractic is that you assess the nervous system, adjust the subluxations you find, and then let the body heal from the inside out—just as the body was designed to do."

In preparation for my assessment during her next visit, I asked Margaret to bring in copies of medical reports as well as a list of drugs that she was taking so we could identify her most serious problems. She arrived for her second appointment with two shopping bags of drugs, as well as a large stack of x-rays and scans. I greeted her and said, "No, Margaret, I only want the drugs you are *currently* taking, not all these."

Margaret replied abruptly, "These *are* just the drugs I'm taking now." Well, my jaw dropped and I could see we were in for a long-term relationship. The two of us poured the pile of drugs on the adjusting table and started to put the puzzle together.

Margaret was on drugs for her heart condition—including cholesterol-lowering medications. There were drugs for arthritis and analgesics (pain killers) for back pain—as well as muscle relaxants to control muscle spasms. She was on antihistamines for hives and rashes, Valium for anxiety, and "The Pill" for hormonal imbalances and polycystic ovaries. She took several drugs for asthma—some daily and others inhaled episodically when her breathing was stressed. In addition to regular antibiotics for urinary tract and lung infections, she required a separate course of medication *with which to treat the thrush caused by the antibiotics!* I had never imagined so many drugs...for so many illnesses... in one person, especially in someone so young!

Margaret was a large girl, and when she tried to lie on the adjusting table, her back would go into extreme muscle spasms and the screaming would start. Everything hurt, and often she would get stuck where she couldn't move and have to pant until the pain passed. It would take all her stamina and two of our practice staff to help her on and off the adjusting table. It required an extended period of time to adjust her as she could only move a few inches at a time. Sometimes, she would have three or four episodes of cramping that would last five minutes each—during a single visit. On her second appointment, she told me that she "hated life." Severely stressed, she was always nervous and anxious about the prospect of not being able to work. During her adjustments, whenever I touched an area on the low (lumbar) part of her back (L-2), she would instantly become "angry" and overwhelmed.

In spite of these difficulties, Margaret persisted in keeping her appointments. And I persisted in adjusting her through the inevitable screams and nasty verbal abuse. Honestly, I often wondered why she bothered to come at all. For *months*, we had a love-hate relationship while the routine went on week after week after week. One day, I bluntly asked Margaret why she kept coming back as I could see no changes. She told me she thought that I cared enough to persist, while her medical doctors just farmed her out to their colleagues because they, themselves, didn't know what to do.

One breakthrough day, there was a glimmer of hope that pierced the fog of Margaret's agony. After six months of care, she told us her sciatic pain had gone and she could stand with her weight on both feet without reliance on a cane. Furthermore, she reported fewer cramps and was sometimes even "feeling better." On April 1st, 1998, Margaret forgot her appointment—a true "first." Concerned about her wellbeing, we called to check if everything was okay. She explained that she was very excited that she had forgotten, because on a *normal* week, she counted down the days until her next adjustment. She was no longer dealing with so many symptoms and was actually starting to feel *human*.

Over the years, small things changed. Margaret told her medical doctor to wean her off one drug at a time as her health improved. After three years and four months of Chiropractic care—with her cardiologist's reluctant agreement—she stopped taking the last of her heart medications. Two months later, Margaret's menstrual cycle renewed for the first time in more than a decade, and it became a monthly occurrence. Bolstered by her Chiropractic-inspired health improvements, Margaret started to question medicine and what her physicians told her to do.

In due course, Margaret was sent for allergy testing. After all those years, it was finally determined that an anesthetic and latex allergy was the original cause for the heart attacks and the many episodes of anaphylaxis she had endured over the years. Her medical doctors re-tested her and noted improvements in her health that they simply couldn't explain. Eventually her lifelong doctor agreed to take her off the last lot of asthma medication and hormone therapy. *Margaret was drug free! (And still is to this day!!)*

Well, now it is a *joy* to see Margaret. She comes in to our Centre regularly for "tune ups" and occasionally makes special appointments when she is "grumpy" or "in a fog." After adjustments, she often comments, "I can 'see better' and can 'focus'." She realizes that "grumpy" and "sarcastic" are not her normal *healthy* state. Margaret has often told us she believes that without Chiropractic, she would no longer be walking this earth. She is thrilled that she's still *working full time* and earning money to put toward the purchase of a home of her own. She goes on fossicking holidays (the Australian hobby of hunting for bits of gold and semi-precious gems), and brings in her booty to the Centre for "show and tell." Every day, Margaret celebrates her new-found health with these words: "Now that I am *alive*, I want to do some *living*."

Oh yes, there is one more life event worthy of note for this Chiropractic patient: Margaret is engaged to be married.

Tracy Kennedy-Shanks, DC
Kennedy Chiropractic Centre
Toowoomba, Queensland
AUSTRALIA

No Work, No Play, and Too Many Trips to the Bathroom

Several years ago, I had hemorrhagic colitis. I couldn't travel five miles in my car without seeking a restroom to pass mucous and blood.

Then one day, I traveled thirty-five miles one-way to attend a talk by a chiropractor, Dr. Jim Sigafoose. He claimed not to treat conditions, or symptoms, but to correct the nerve interference causing cellular dysfunction throughout the body.

He explained that the brain stem controls all of the body's physiology, and pressure on the stem from the first bone in the neck may contribute to the problem.

He talked about an "Innate Intelligence" that contributes to survival, adaptation, replication, reproduction, and does the healing—when expressed through the cells of the body.

He advised I be x-rayed, scanned, and adjusted, if necessary, then checked on a regular basis to determine the need for an adjustment that day.

He suggested I eat more than baby food and mush—that sounded good, since I had lost 68 pounds in a year.

Trying to run a print shop, I couldn't work, play, or do much else—other than attend the bathroom.

Four days after my first adjustment, I had the first formed bowel movement in ages, slept all night, had no cramps, and woke up in the morning knowing that all would be well.

It took eight months for me to regain my normal weight, but I was working and living a normal life within a few months.

Today, all is well, and my wife and I still see the chiropractor for regular adjustments. Except, now we see his daughter, who carries on his practice after he retired to travel and do seminars.

The one thing that sticks in my mind is when he said, "I don't treat symptoms or disease, I correct nerve interference, and the power that made the body heals the body."

Ralph Johnson
Grateful former patient of
Jim Sigafoose, DC
Sigafoose Seminars
Aberdeen, Maryland

Dr. Sigafoose is the author of
Good Medicine

9

I Got My Life Back!

"Birds sing after a storm; why shouldn't people feel as free to delight in whatever remains to them?"

Rose Fitzgerald Kennedy
Mother of nine children including
President John F. Kennedy,
Senator Robert F. Kennedy, and
Senator Edward M. Kennedy
(1890-1995)

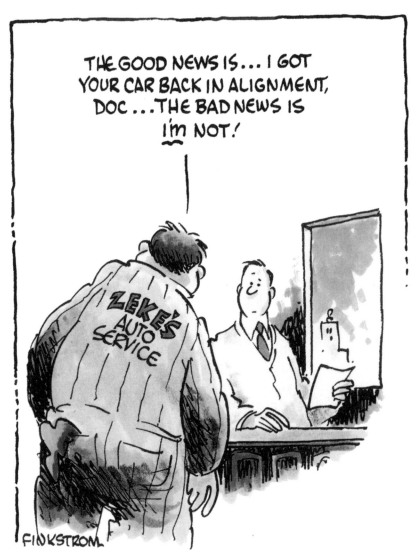

Reprinted by arrangement with Finkstrom Licensing International

The Hidden Power of a Chiropractic Adjustment

Back in 1995, one of our longtime patients was telling her friend, Rosie, how pleased she was with the care she received at our practice. Soon afterward, Rosie's husband called and scheduled a consultation for his wife.

On the morning of Rosie's appointment, the plate glass door to our office swung open wide and a large lady—weighing at least 350 pounds—entered the reception area. Dressed in a soiled, full-length nightshirt, she had to shuffle in sideways to clear the door. A somewhat smaller man, obviously Rosie's husband, was doing his best to prop up his wife as she inched her way toward the front desk.

Rosie's appearance caused every patient in the reception area to avert their eyes so as not to be caught staring. Moments later, however, another sense was assaulted: the room was filled with an extremely unpleasant *smell!* Personal hygiene was, unfortunately, another casualty in Rosie's daily war on pain.

Georgia, our receptionist, quickly stepped out from behind the front desk and greeted the couple, "Good morning; how can we help you?"

Rosie, the expression on her face making clear that she was in enormous pain, introduced herself. Overwhelmed with compassion for Rosie's discomfort, Georgia led the pair to one of our two private consultation rooms. Rosie was given a seat on the padded, steel-framed, Leander adjusting table while her husband was seated on one of the two chairs along the wall. Georgia then had my assistant confer with Rosie and complete a health history. As soon as the paperwork was finished, my assistant advised me that we had a special case requiring my immediate attention.

When I entered Rosie's consultation room, I found a lady in her mid-thirties whose beautiful face was contorted in pain and anguish. After I introduced myself, I asked her how we could be of service. Here is what I learned.

Rosie had been medically diagnosed with varying degrees of pain since early childhood. For 27 years, she had been subjected to an increasingly complex, and ever-more-powerful, array of pharmaceuticals—none of which provided more than temporary relief.

To make matters worse, for the previous three years her condition had escalated to—and was medically diagnosed as—fibromyalgia plus possible *reflex sympathetic dystrophy* (RSD). Rosie described her condition as excruciating pain—twenty-four hours a day—and her medical doctors had given her a very poor prognosis. Medical translation: "Learn to live with it; take your meds; there is no cure!"

Rosie explained that, with the onset of fibromyalgia plus possible RSD, she rapidly started putting on weight due to the new, more-powerful medications and subsequent lack of energy. She could only manage to get a couple of hours' sleep in every twenty-four! Constantly restless, she spent all of her time in bed praying for the blessing of sleep. Not long after being slammed with her worsened condition, she was no longer able to complete her responsibilities at work and had to quit her job—a job that had previously given her enormous satisfaction, enabled her to contribute to the family's finances, and bolstered her self-esteem.

When Rosie was finished, she asked, "Dr. Mancini, do you think Chiropractic can help me?" I told her that I would need to perform a comprehensive exam before answering her question.

I continued by explaining that, in our practice, more than 80 percent of the patients we accepted got well from Chiropractic.

I then proceeded to give Rosie a full physical exam including orthopedic and neurological testing, checking her cranial nerves, taking x-rays, and palpating her spine and the rest of her skeletal structure. I discovered nerve interferences (subluxations causing pinched nerves) throughout her spine. After finishing, I presented her and her husband with my Report of Findings, explained that I was willing to accept her case, and that it would be my pleasure to welcome her as our newest patient. Rosie's treatment began the following day.

Adjusting Rosie was a challenge due to her obesity and the fact that she was in such great discomfort. Every time I had to move a part of her body, she cried out in pain. For a typical treatment—with the help of her husband, I'd assist Rosie onto the table face down. I would then administer a variety of Chiropractic adjustments to remove neural interferences so that her body could start to heal naturally.

For the first couple of weeks, I saw her daily. For the next four weeks, she was treated three times weekly. At that point, she had experienced tremendous improvement—about 80 percent. She reported that she was able to resume a normal life; and we performed a formal progress evaluation. Adjusting her became much easier since her pain was greatly reduced. (One of the more subtle indicators of progress is that her personal hygiene improved dramatically!) Following my recommendation for continuing care, she started coming in twice a week. A couple of months after that, the frequency of her treatment was reduced to once a week.

After six months, Rosie tearfully announced that her husband's company was transferring him to a different state. She said she would really miss the compassionate care she had come to associate with our entire staff. Of course, I was more than happy to assist her in locating a chiropractor not far from her new home.

About a year after I became president of the Parker College of Chiropractic, my administrative assistant buzzed me on the intercom and said, "Dr. Mancini, there's a lady named Rosie calling for you who says she's one of your old patients."

I said to myself, "Rosie? Could this be the *same* Rosie?"

I answered the phone and Rosie said, "Dr. Mancini, I just heard that you were leading Parker College, and I wanted to say, 'Congratulations!' "

"Rosie," I said, "I'm doing great! How are you?"

"Oh, Dr. Mancini, I've been losing weight—more than 175 pounds so far! I feel like I have my life back. I have a great job. Everything is wonderful!"

"That's terrific! I'm so happy for you, Rosie."

"But you know, Dr. Mancini, I really wanted to call primarily because I never thanked you; and I also never told you something I'm about to tell you now."

"What is it, Rosie? You know, it was *my* pleasure to take care of *you!*"

"Well, you remember when I first came into your office; you saw the shape I was in? You could tell I wasn't very happy; I was deeply depressed. What I didn't tell you is that my husband had told me two weeks before that he was going to divorce me. He said that every time he tried to get close to me, I would push him away. Every time that he needed something from me, I wasn't there for him. He was actually raising the kids by himself and working full-time just to keep the household going.

"You remember my children—aged five, eight, and ten at the time? They totally *hated* me!"

"What do you mean, Rosie?"

"Every time my children wanted to play with me, I couldn't because of my pain. Every time they wanted me to hug them, I couldn't, so they thought I didn't love them. I couldn't put them to bed; I couldn't help them with their homework; I couldn't be supportive of them. I was in bed all the time—angry, upset, and constantly feeling guilty.

"Right before I saw you the first time, I thought, 'I'm losing my husband, I've lost my children, I've lost my job. What do I have to live for? I have *nothing* to live for!'

"What I desperately needed was HOPE! And that's what you gave me! No other healthcare practitioner had offered me the kind of hope I was looking for before I visited your office. When you said that our bodies were able to heal themselves, I'd never heard that from any other physician or doctor. When you told me that the main objective of Chiropractic is to remove the interferences preventing the body from healing itself, it just made perfect sense to me."

Then she said something for which I was *totally* unprepared, "Dr. Mancini, what I didn't tell you is that just two days before I first saw you, I bought a gun. I'd already made up my mind that I would kill myself if I didn't feel that you or Chiropractic could help me. *I just want to thank you for saving my life!*"

I froze. I couldn't believe what I was hearing. When I reflected on what she said, it made me recognize that we chiropractors usually have no idea the impact we have on people's lives. Yes, we know that people recover from their pain. Sometimes we know that they get back to their regular activities: work, golf, travel, or whatever their life pursuits may be.

But it's rare that a patient shares with us the deep impact of Chiropractic care such as averting a possible divorce, improving the relationship with their children, being able to resume work, but most amazing of all, the prospect of saving someone from suicide by removing their misery.

That's when I recognized that the power of a Chiropractic adjustment is so much *more* than we give it credit for. It impacts everyone's life physically, mentally, and spiritually. *That* is the reason why—every single day—I do what I do with the understanding that we have a world that is deserving of being able to actually live life to the fullest. I believe Chiropractic supports every individual to do that—to maximize their *health potential* so they can maximize their *life potential!*

Fabrizio Mancini, DC
President
Parker College of Chiropractic
Dallas, Texas
As told to Don Dible

No More Migraines!

My name is Sandy, and I'm forty-three-years old. Since I was seventeen, I've suffered from severe migraines. From that point on in my life, I always knew that I'd be in bed at least three or four times a month—completely debilitated with all the symptoms that go with migraines: vomiting, sensitivity to light and noise, and the feeling of wishing I could chop off my head and put it in the freezer. No joke—anyone with migraines knows *exactly* what I'm talking about!

"You have to learn how to live with it," my family said. It was genetic, they told me; and it was inevitable, because my mother and several aunts and cousins all had the same problem. So, despite trying Western medicine, homeopathic remedies, and many other things, I "lived with it" for more than twenty-five years!

One day, when I was going for my gym routine—one of those rare days when I didn't have a headache, I saw a sign posted about an evening seminar on migraines. I remember thinking, "How bad can it be? I've tried everything else; I have nothing to lose."

So that night, I went to the seminar and met Dr. Brad Pennington. His seminar was very informative about the cause and effects of migraines, and he indicated that many migraine-sufferers benefit from Chiropractic care. I remember thinking, "Wow, what a bold statement!" But then, again, I thought, "What I have I got to lose?" Even though I was very skeptical—who wouldn't be after 25 years of migraines, I signed up for my first consultation.

That was the beginning of a new life for me. Writing this story, I feel a little emotional and teary, because Dr. Brad truly changed my world. He put me on a program of Chiropractic treatment. He explained everything extremely well with examples, drawings, and handouts. At first, I saw Dr. Brad several times a week. Over time, the frequency of my adjustments was reduced to the "maintenance level" of once a month. The results were almost immediately noticeable. For the first time in my life, I didn't have to take time off from work, or spend my days off in bed. *For the first time in my life, I didn't have to be afraid of my body and what it would or wouldn't do!*

The revelation is that I can now trust my body to be healthy! I can do *anything—at any time*—without pain or fear of what's coming. Yes, choosing Chiropractic was a commitment. Yes, it was scary. And yes, it was worth every penny and every minute. *Nothing can describe the gratitude I have for the talented, gifted hands of my chiropractor and love with which my adjustments are administered.* Dr. Brad believes in what he does and it shows. With monthly maintenance, my body stays tuned and healthy. Not only are the migraines gone, but I'm overall much healthier. I am rarely sick, and my stamina has improved enormously.

So, for anyone out there that still has doubts, I am proof it works! I feel alive! Go for it; do it! Take control over your body and health now, it is worth it!

Sandy Jacobs
Chiropractic advocate and
Grateful patient of
Brad Pennington, DC
Denver Chiropractic
Denver, Colorado

How I Discovered True Wellness

The Métis people are the descendants of marriages of Inuit, Ojibway, Algonquin, Cree, Saulteau, Menomineee, and other indigenous Canadian peoples to Europeans and other ethnicities from all over the world. In Canada, they are officially recognized as aboriginal peoples and live in cooperatives in much the same way as their counterparts in the United States live on reservations. Today, living conditions on these cooperatives are similar to what is typically found in Third World countries. Poverty is commonplace and the health of the general population is uniformly dismal.

I was born to a fourteen-year old Métis child-mother who had the foresight to see that life in a cooperative would not be best for her new offspring. My mother gave me the most wonderful gift possible—at great sacrifice to her maternal instinct.

She put me up for adoption.

I spent my first three months in foster care before I was placed with my adoptive parents—the good people whom today I call "family."

As far back as I can remember, my health was always precarious. I recall that, as a child, I was given awful-tasting, iron-fortified black syrup to treat my anemia. I also remember being told what a great baby I was—I slept for very long periods of time. Throughout childhood, I was always underweight. At about nine-years of age, my tonsils were removed and I hemorrhaged profusely. Since my anemic blood refused to clot, I had to be cauterized numerous times during the surgery or I would have bled to death. As I emerged from the general anesthetic, my heart rate escalated to an alarming level before returning to normal. My adoptive mother was summoned to the recovery room because the hospital staff thought I might not survive.

From a very young age, I remember believing that "sickness" was my natural state. As I grew older, I solidified that "victim" mentality. Every physician I saw asked about my genetic predisposition to disease. And every time that question was posed, I shrank a little more into my sickness belief system. I simply didn't have any information about what my genetic potential actually was.

Throughout my high school years, my sicknesses continued. I got every "normal" illness you can imagine including colds, flu, impetigo, etc. At one point, a physician diagnosed my "illness *du jour*" as chronic fatigue syndrome or CFS. This clinical observation came as no surprise to me! The "perfect" sleeping baby was now a teenager—exhausted all the time "for no apparent reason." Although I dutifully enrolled in the academically-required physical education classes, I always had to drop out due to poor health. I failed every Canadian fitness test I ever took. I couldn't even do the 800-meter run around the track. Nor could I engage my lower-lumbar spine and core to execute a *single* sit-up.

When I was sixteen, I started to notice large lumps on my lumbar spine (low back) and was unable to get up in the morning without intense pain and stiffness. My mother took me to a physician who x-rayed my spine and then told me that I was born missing one of the lower vertebrae. He said nothing could be done to remedy the problem except to take more medication.

At the age of nineteen, I was diagnosed with cancer of the cervix. In due course, I was treated with the standard regimen of surgery, radiation, and chemotherapy. That completed, I was pronounced "in remission."

At twenty-one, my bladder and kidneys started "failing." (I didn't even know they had taken a test!) Following painful, invasive, diagnostic procedures, no cause could be determined.

In the classic medical tradition, I was told to continue taking anti-inflammatory drugs, auto-immune suppressants, and antibiotics. The physicians said they were unable to find anything "wrong," so they could not prescribe a more effective treatment.

I was in my mid-twenties when I first experienced Chiropractic care. Prior to that time, I had had no contact with chiropractors or Chiropractic patients. In fact, I had vague misgivings about Chiropractic due to simple ignorance. What little I *thought* I knew about it proved to be wrong. As I started to discover the body's inborn ability to heal itself, I began to reject my previous acceptance of sickness as a normal state. I made a conscious decision to reject the three nervous system stressors that were keeping me in a constant state of sickness. Chemically, I was dependent on antibiotics, pain killers, and digestive medication. Physically, I was never active enough to turn off my stressors. And emotionally, I was always exhausted and withdrawn—unable to "engage" life.

Having discovered Chiropractic care, I started attending lectures by leaders in the profession. They introduced me to the vital roles that a positive attitude and a properly-functioning nervous system play in regulating health and wellness. My health improvement happened over such a long period of time—and so gradually—that it was almost unnoticeable. By far the largest change I experienced was in my *attitude*. After that got "adjusted," everything else improved in perfect harmony. I began to see the possibility of a healthy future. At 28-years of age, I started running. Ten months later, I ran an ultra-marathon in the mountains. I have since run four half-marathons. I've discontinued antibiotics as well as digestive medication and have been drug-free for a full seven-years-and-counting.

Each morning, I wake up and ask myself, "What I can do today to sustain and feed my soul?" Every day, I expect more of myself and more of my health. I no longer think of sickness as my constant companion. In fact, sickness and I have gone our separate ways—permanently! I always encourage others to achieve more of their health potential. At a time when people in the wealthiest countries of the world are dying at alarming rates, something needs to change. I believe we all need to change our attitude about health, our willingness to do something about it, and put Chiropractic at center stage.

My decision to consciously reject sickness as a way of life is not unique. All I had at my disposal was a little more information than the average person and a desire to be TRULY well. True wellness lies at the *heart* of Chiropractic philosophy. Nothing more, nothing less.

Brandi MacDonald
President
True Concepts Inc.
Edmonton, Alberta
CANADA

Disappearing Psoriasis

I cannot remember a time when my parents were not receiving Chiropractic care. As a child, I followed their example of being a patient without questioning the importance of my actions. Thus, at 17 years of age, I didn't understand the consequences of receiving a Chiropractic adjustment and let school and work get in the way of scheduling a visit. The occasional trips to the chiropractor's office were in times of pain—specifically knee pain that had developed.

A few years later, as the manager of a convenience store, I was overworked and exhausted. The amount of stress that crushed me every day was at its pinnacle and difficult to bear. It was a result of dealing with employees under my direction, some of whom sometimes came to work under the influence of narcotics, working in an area that was socio-economically underprivileged, and having to cope with the constant presence of thieves and police in the store and its surroundings. Physical symptoms of stress began to develop: emotional outbursts, sleep deprivation, tremors, migraines, gastro-intestinal difficulties, chronic tonsillitis and sinusitis, panic attacks, and agoraphobia. Additionally, I saw psoriasis develop on 80% of my body. Medications, including antibiotics, made their place in my daily diet.

It's when I went to the bank one day that my life changed, as I noticed that the Chiropractic clinic next door was in need of a receptionist. My lifestyle was in desperate need of change, and I took the opportunity that seemed to be offering itself to me. A quick phone call to the chiropractor who owns the clinic led me to being offered the job a week later, one which I most graciously accepted, and which marked the beginning of my true experience with Chiropractic.

Soon after becoming Dr. Renée Dallaire's new assistant, I also became her patient. When she observed the psoriasis that covered most of my body, Dr. Dallaire took my medical history. During the initial consultation, she had me undergo a complete exam that included taking a number of x-rays. She then explained what, exactly, this beautiful profession is all about.

During a subsequent visit, Dr. Dallaire took the time to provide further explanations of the human nervous system and how the human body reacts to different changes in spinal alignment. I was extremely fascinated by all the information she presented and discovered the awe-inspiring machinery that is the human body. For the first time in my life, I understood the importance of a Chiropractic adjustment.

The first week of care was the most difficult. One morning, I had to call in sick because it was next to impossible for me to get out of bed. I had major symptoms of gastroenteritis. My call to Dr. Dallaire that morning was difficult for me as I had to tell her that I was physically incapable of going to work.

Her explanation on the process of detoxification of the body left me sceptical; however I soon realized that she was correct as I saw and felt the symptoms of my ailment decrease and come to disappear as the morning approached noon. To aid me in my attempt to sleep and get over any sickness, Dr. Dallaire suggested I make my way to her office for an adjustment as soon as possible.

In continuing with Chiropractic care on a regular basis, I soon observed a difference in my daily life. After about a year-and-a-half, the migraines that had resulted from the stress of my former job had completely disappeared. The next thing to change was the psoriasis. Around 60% of the disease that affected my skin was eliminated, and I was ecstatic to see it leave. Antibiotics are now a thing of the past and have been for about three-and-a-half years, along with the chronic sinusitis and tonsillitis to which I had been accustomed.

The overall quality of my life has greatly improved, and my experience with Chiropractic has taught me to be more aware of my body. Thanks to Chiropractic, my life has completely changed for the better and I continue to see positive change daily.

As I reflect on the condition of my life four years ago, I thank heaven for the great gift of Chiropractic. I must admit that Chiropractic affects more than just your physical health; it is critical to having and maintaining a healthy physical and psychological lifestyle. With Dr. Dallaire's help, I have not only come to respect and listen to my body, but also put words on my thoughts and channel my negative emotions in order to ease my walk through life. Through the channel of my work and in my personal life, I am constantly sharing my positive experience with Chiropractic. It is my deepest belief that all should know about and experience this astonishing profession. As for me, Chiropractic has become an integral part of my lifestyle recognizing that a healthy spine and nervous system are essential to living the healthy life you desire.

Annick Fecteau
Chiropractic advocate and
Grateful patient of
Renée Dallaire, DC
Centre Chiropratique Des Sources
Pointe-Claire, Québec
CANADA

Adult Onset Puberty

After graduating from college in 1985, I joined the Peace Corps to see the world and, like most of my Corps colleagues, to figure out what I wanted to do with the rest of my life. My first assignment was in sunny Belize, Central America, where—after four months of service as a high school chemistry teacher—I was hit by a tortilla truck while walking to class along the side of a dirt road.

Air-ambulanced to a hospital in sunny Florida, I spent three weeks in a coma. When I awoke, I had no short-term memory. Having regained consciousness, I was transferred to a new home—a head-injury rehabilitation center in snowy, mid-winter Boston, near where my family lived. No palm trees there!

My immediate reality was that I couldn't walk or talk; my entire right side was paralyzed; and the nurses had taken my glasses. Since I'm legally blind without my glasses, I was *not* a happy camper!

For the next year, I received physical, occupational, and speech therapy. At that point, I could kind of walk, kind of move my right arm, and—*whee*—*talk* again! However, the hospital—a dumping ground for individuals too damaged by neurological injuries to ever return to any kind of normal existence—was rather depressing. The "know-it-all" staff MDs informed my parents that I could look forward to nothing better than a lifetime in institutions. I *strongly* disagreed, and wasted no time in formulating an "escape plan"!

The Boston area is home to many renowned colleges and universities, so I pored over various catalogs and chose a course on brain integration and growth at Boston College—easily reached by public transportation with the aid of my walker. (Having graduated pre-med, I'd already taken the prerequisites.) Although the course wasn't too exciting, it proved to me that academia was still an option. However, medical school was no longer of interest to me given the attitude of the majority of MDs I'd encountered toward brain injuries and "less-than-perfect" individuals.

Glowing from the success of having passed the Boston College course, but still blocked from further progress by the MDs and hospital administrators, it was time for me to pull out the heavy artillery—help from outsiders who might be concerned. This took the form of letters to the high school principal of Muffles College in Belize, the directors of the Peace Corps in Central America, and—last-but-not-least, the President of the United States! After a seemingly interminable wait, permission was finally granted and hospital discharge papers were issued.

I believe in finishing what I start, so I returned to Belize and the high school in which I'd been teaching before the "tortilla truck interruption" or "TTI." A Belize neighbor took one look at me and—due to my obviously unstable gait and difficulty with the most mundane tasks—suggested I come along on her biweekly visits to the one chiropractor in the entire country. How exciting; I'd never been to a chiropractor before! After my first eight-hour bus ride, one-way, to his office, and my first Chiropractic adjustment, I discovered that this man and his healing art held the key to helping my damaged body function better! I continued to see him for the rest of the time I was in Belize. It was during my stay in that lovely country that I discovered what I wanted to do with the rest of my life: become a chiropractor! Thank you, Peace Corps!

While I was in Chiropractic College, a fellow student (soon to become my husband) told me about this "special" doctor he wanted me to see. Since I'd had such a fantastic experience with Chiropractic in Belize, I enthusiastically embraced the idea.

Although I was still recovering from the TTI five years before, I was sufficiently functional to attend Chiropractic College but was far from being in optimal shape. My residual brain injury symptom was the post-concussive fog in which I'd been living ever since—apparent to others; not so obvious to me. While I could function day-to-day and pass exams in school, I didn't have a clear notion of where I fit in time-and-space. I was, to put it bluntly, "out of it."

My fiancée dragged me more than 400 miles to see this "special" chiropractor he'd heard about. The doctor studied x-rays of my head and neck and then lined me up on his adjusting table. He gave me an imperceptible impulse to my upper neck and I screamed!

Not to worry; it didn't hurt. The sudden release from the fog I'd been living under for five years was immediate and complete! I was overwhelmed, hence the scream. And I was able to instantly remember what I had felt like before the accident. I hadn't even realized I was only half-living ever since the TTI.

There's a great deal more to my story than that moment, however. When I was born, I experienced some type of trauma, and I'd grown up with that. As a result, some nerve connections had never fully developed. Not until I was 27 years old did I finally get those nerve interferences fixed! That's the only conclusion I can come to when—within the next three months—I "finished" puberty. I thought I'd completed that a decade and a half earlier.

I discovered that some of my shoes were suddenly too small as my feet grew more than half a size. Also, during those three months, all my pants quickly grew too short for me. And my breasts grew more than a size larger! The most dramatic change, however, was when I woke up one morning and discovered I could see 3-dimensionally FOR THE FIRST TIME IN MY LIFE. Since I was born, I'd only looked out of one eye. As a child, my dominant eye had been patched every year so my weaker one could get stronger. As a result, I became accustomed to looking through just one eye to see. Suddenly, I was observing the world with *both* of my eyes simultaneously. W-O-W, I can't begin to describe the difference! I spent the next two days in bed, trying to get used to this new sensation.

Needless to say, I am today a chiropractor—as is my husband. We specialize in the treatment of nerve damage and interference. Occasionally, we have the good fortune to unleash dramatic changes in our patients. Life is good!

Dorrin B. Rosenfeld, DC
State of the Art Chiropractic
Vallejo, California

10

Surgery? Just Say No!

"Surgery is always second best.
If you can do something else, it's better."

John W. Kirklin, MD
While at the Mayo Clinic, Dr. Kirklin performed the world's
first series of open-heart operations using a heart-lung machine.
(1917-2004)

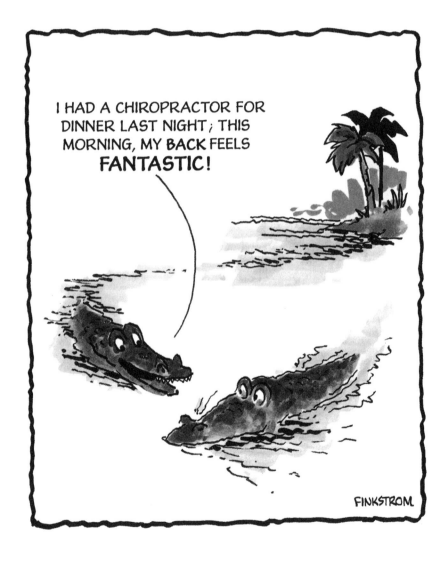

Chiropractic Saved My Life!

When I received my Doctor of Chiropractic degree in 1979, I dedicated my life to the wellbeing of others. You can imagine my humble satisfaction when, year after year, delighted patients regularly referred relatives, friends, and co-workers to the office. By the end of my first twelve months of practice—and for the next 24 years—I had the pleasure of seeing hundreds of patients every week!

Now, it's a fact that no dedicated doctor wants to refuse care to any patient—especially if he or she can help them achieve complete health and wellness. Rather than limit my practice, I accepted anyone who needed my care. In the fullness of time, I found myself working ten or more hours a day—all week long. Not surprisingly, after more than two decades, my own health had begun to suffer as I placed the needs of my patients ahead of my own. Although I knew better—I had benefitted from Chiropractic care since I was a boy of twelve—the most I allowed myself was probably one or two adjustments a month. Typically, it was less.

Not until 2003 did I finally accept the fact I was desperately ill. My symptoms? Shortness of breath, constant fatigue, and dizziness with even the slightest exertion. These problems had begun years before, but all I had done was curtail my activities. An avid runner for many years, I stopped running and put a halt to all my sports activities. By the time I admitted my failing health, I couldn't walk 100 feet without gasping for air. Traversing a simple flight of stairs was sheer torture. In the evenings, on returning home, I'd often have to stop once or twice on the driveway while walking the short distance from my car to the front porch.

Early on, I attributed my discomfort to allergies. To remove allergens from my environment, I began with our home heating and air conditioning system where I had all the duct work professionally cleaned and expensive filters installed. I even went so far as to have the indoor swimming pool drained and cleaned—again, by a professional. (There would be no more chlorine in our home!) But my symptoms persisted. In order to continue adjusting patients, I made use of a Ventolin® rescue inhaler, sucking aerosol-driven albuterol sulfate into my lungs every 30 to 45 minutes each day during my adjusting time!

Following a comprehensive exam, my cardiologist announced his diagnosis: Primary Pulmonary Hypertension (PPH). Any way you pronounce them, the combination of those three words doesn't sound good. One of the insidious characteristics of this disease is that it develops very slowly. As a result, it's often *years* before victims realize they're sick. Yup! That's *exactly* what happened to me.

PPH is a blood reflux, of sorts. The right ventricle in my heart was trying to pump blood into my lungs; but—according to the results of an echocardiogram—the back pressure was as much as 57 millimeters of mercury instead of the normal 15! In other words, my lungs were unable to oxygenate my blood; that's why I was constantly out of breath. I had no back pain, no neck pain. As a matter of fact, I had no pain anywhere; I just could not *breathe*! That's why it took me years to accept the fact I was *sick*!

What my cardiologist urged next *really* took my breath away: A DOUBLE LUNG AND HEART TRANSPLANT!

Now, I've always been faithful to the Chiropractic lifestyle. For me, a double lung and heart transplant simply was not an option! I concluded that if my transition was supposed to happen; then that's God's way of telling me my time here on Earth is done. So be it. Spiritually, I was okay with that!

I spent the next six months searching for two caring chiropractors to take over my practice. When I found them, I retired—fully expecting to die in the subsequent twelve to eighteen months as forecast by my cardiologist. You could say that—as of April 15, 2004—I turned my back on Chiropractic's adjusting tables. Considering the fact I was born in 1955—you do the math—I was still a young man!

About a month later, I awoke one morning with an epiphany—as though I had been hit over the head with a metaphorical sledge-hammer. I thought to myself, "You idiot! You've been preaching Chiropractic for 25 years; you tell anybody who will listen about nervous system integrity. There's gotta' be something wrong with your *spine* that's affecting the nervous system that governs your lungs and your heart!" As today's teenagers might say, "Like, WOW, man; what a *concept!*"

In no time at all, I scheduled a complete Chiropractic examination. It turned out I had a *beautiful* spine! At least *parts* of it were beautiful. My neck had a nice, normal-forward curvature; my lumbar spine had a normal curvature; I even had a nice, level pelvis. BUT—from the seventh cervical to the fourth thoracic vertebra—my spine was a complete mess. And what area do you think supplies the heart and the lungs? C-7 to T-4!

Starting in late May, I faithfully reported to my chiropractor for daily adjustments. Within a month, I realized that I was able to walk with no shortness of breath. By the end of August, the three-mile trek to my cardiologist's Toronto office—on foot—was accomplished with no shortness of breath whatsoever. My scheduled echocardiogram revealed a drop in pulmonary pressure to 27—down significantly from the previous reading of 57!

Troubled by this astounding drop—achieved without the benefit of his prescribed surgical intervention—my cardiologist was seriously convinced there had been an error in the diagnostic procedure. Later that day, I submitted to a second echocardiogram. Secretly, I already knew in my heart what was wrong with the first echocardiogram—ABSOLUTELY NOTHING!

The rest is history. What's my pulmonary pressure now? I don't know, and I don't care. I'm healthy, I work out, and I get adjusted every single week without fail. Obviously, I haven't gone back to seeing 100 or more patients a day; that part of my life is over. A new chapter has begun; a new door has opened for me.

What's so gratifying about my life now is that I'm still able to follow my passion! Today, I serve my beloved profession as a vice president at the Parker College of Chiropractic where I'm in charge of seminars—with the help of a fabulous, fabulous team. My responsibilities also include service as Vice President of Development and Alumni Relations (fundraising—a vital function in any academic institution). At Parker, our declared mission is to serve Chiropractic *worldwide*; and every day, I give thanks for the opportunity to help the College achieve that objective!

Before taking on my current duties, I had spent years serving Parker as a speaker. When my appointment was announced, most folks in the profession who knew me said, "Gilles, this is a natural; you were *called* to become the Director of Parker Seminars."

As I reflect on these events, I'm fascinated by one simple question: "Did I develop primary pulmonary hypertension because I was supposed to *transition*...to the Parker College of Chiropractic?"

Without the trauma of PPH, I would never have left the patients whom I dearly loved, and I would never have retired from Chiropractic practice. Literally, until the PPH detour, I expected to die someday "with my boots on"—at the age of 85-95-100, whatever it would be—adjusting a patient. But God had different plans for me; and here I am...at Parker.

Gilles A. LaMarche, DC
Vice President
Parker College of Chiropractic
Dallas, Texas

ZZZZZZZZZZZZZ!

Our family has a new appreciation for the benefits of Chiropractic. Although we haven't received regular care, my husband and I have both had adjustments at different times throughout our adult lives. Until recently, we never thought of taking our children—three boys—in for adjustments.

Four weeks ago, I was discussing my son, Zachary, with a friend who suggested that I take him to see Dr. Wilson. She told me that he was her chiropractor and that he worked with children. I was tired and frustrated and felt that I had nothing to lose, so I made an appointment.

Zachary, our oldest, is seven. Except for insomnia, he's been a relatively healthy child—troubled only by normal childhood illnesses such as asthma, allergies, and occasional colds. But Zachary has always had problems sleeping. He only slept through the night a few times in his entire life. He snores loudly and has sleep apnea. He's had these problems since he was only a few months old. Then, he was diagnosed with sleep apnea by two different pediatricians. I've discussed Zachary's sleeping problems with his pediatricians throughout the years.

When Zachary had his first birthday, I took him in for his well baby check. I talked to the doctor about how much he woke up at night and how exhausted I was. He told me that Zachary had formed some bad habits and that I needed to let him cry. My husband and I tried this, but it was not successful. Zachary would cry himself to sleep, but wake up again a short time later. He normally got up about seven times a night.

Finally, the doctor prescribed Atarax, a potent antihistamine often used to treat insomnia. He told me to give Zachary a teaspoonful at bedtime. This didn't help Zachary sleep one bit better. When we moved to Albuquerque and started to see a new pediatrician, I discussed Zachary's frequent waking at night with her. She discussed behavioral modification techniques and suggested giving him Benadryl, another antihistamine, before bedtime. She said the snoring was because his tonsils and adenoids were too large and that they should be removed when he turned five.

Zachary's problem was not failure to go to bed at a reasonable hour. He'd go to bed and fall asleep easily. It's just that he woke up every couple of hours and snored so loudly you could hear him from the other side of the house. He was two-years of age at this point.

Zachary continued to grow and do reasonably well in spite of the fact that he never slept soundly. We began to think that he was just a child who didn't require much sleep and that he would always snore. I always discussed his sleep patterns with the doctor at his annual checkups. I've received lots of different advice and medications. Nothing seemed to make a difference.

This year, Zachary is seven. He has continued to have the same difficulties sleeping; he rarely sleeps through the night. It makes me nervous to sleep with him because you can watch him stop breathing for several seconds and then gasp for air. He still snores very loudly. Our doctor has attributed his snoring and frequent waking to allergies. He had Zachary on Zyrtec, albuterol, and two different steroid-based nasal sprays daily. Even on all of this medication, Zachary's sleep problems have persisted. We've cycled him on and off these medications many times through the years.

I became very concerned this year because Zachary's second grade teacher has called several times to say that he was falling asleep in class. His snoring and poor sleep habits have become worse. He was getting up and waking me every few hours. One night, he got up fifteen times! We were both exhausted the next morning. It didn't matter how early he went to bed, he still looked tired in the morning. He always had dark circles under his eyes.

We've had his eyes checked four times in the last two years because he's always complaining of headaches. I was afraid there was something seriously wrong with him. The final straw was when his school nurse called me at work to say that I was an irresponsible mother for not making him go to bed earlier at night. I was frustrated and angry. I picked him up from school and took him straight to the doctor's office. I was told to take him off all medications once again; and we would slowly reintroduce them because one of them may be making him sleepy. The doctor also recommended that we have several tests such as a swallow study, a CAT scan, and x-rays. He also said that Zachary's tonsils and adenoids would have to come out.

This is the point we were at when I met Dr. Wilson. We had decided to go ahead and have his tonsils removed because several different doctors through the years had recommended this. We felt desperate because Zachary's schooling was being affected. He simply couldn't continue to sleep through classes at school. He was always tired and irritable in the evenings.

Dr. Wilson scanned Zachary's spine and found several areas that were out of alignment. He recommended that we bring Zachary in for several visits. After Zachary's second adjustment, he slept through the night. I thought it was just a coincidence, but he has continued to do well. Zachary has slept through the night *every* night since that second visit. Although he still snores, it is only an occasional *light* snore. *I* haven't slept this well in *his* life.

Zachary's teacher called me last week to let me know that she had noticed a major change in his behavior at school. She didn't know that we have been taking him to the chiropractor. She said that he had energy now that she had not seen all year. He was no longer lethargic. He used to always put his head down on his desk during class. She said he had quit doing that and hadn't fallen asleep once. He hasn't complained of any more headaches and has more energy at night. I also have more energy, because I'm also getting more sleep. We've canceled the surgery to remove his tonsils and have taken him off all medications. I've been so thrilled with the results of Zachary's treatment that I'm also taking my other two children for Chiropractic care with Dr. Wilson.

Jennifer Smith
Chiropractic advocate
Mother of Zachary Smith,
A happy, healthy patient of
T. D. Wilson, DC
Global Health Chiropractic
Lubbock, Texas

How I Avoided Neck Surgery

Hello, my name is Lori Dahl, and I'm 41-years old. I've always been very athletic; and, until last February, I never thought *anything* could stop me from participating in recreational activities.

Last winter, my husband and I resumed skiing after a fifteen-year hiatus. While I didn't take any dramatic falls, a couple of days later I noticed that my right hand was tingling. Soon after that, I developed numbness in the same hand.

Then the *pain* started—BIG TIME! First, in my right elbow, then it traveled up to my shoulder with massive shooting pains down my whole right side.

Yes, I thought the pain would go away—eventually. But as the months dragged on, I became more and more debilitated. I could no longer sleep on my right side, and was having trouble sitting in one position on *any* kind of chair for more than a couple of minutes! Trust me: No matter *what* your health problem is, sleep-deprivation is guaranteed to make it worse!

When I was in almost more pain than I could stand, a very athletic colleague at work (who doesn't believe in Chiropractic in any way, shape, or form) insisted that I see his physician. This jock bragged that his orthopedist was "the best sports medicine doctor" he'd ever seen. So, off I went, hoping and praying that my work-buddy's doc would "cure" me.

After several visits, the orthopedist had me taking Lortabs and Percoset for pain. I was also taking an anti-inflammatory drug plus being injected with Novocain-laced-cortisone. (Now, there's a *nasty* cocktail!) All of these worked great—as Band-Aids. When their effects wore off, the pain would just come back... with a *vengeance!*

All the while, the orthopedist was telling me that—on a scale of 1-5 in severity of degeneration of the 6th and 7th disks in my neck, I was between a 3 and a 4. Of course, that diagnosis made me feel a whole lot better, right? NOT! The only medical remedy he proposed: SURGERY! In the meantime, he wanted me to see a neurologist who would determine the extent of my nerve damage and get a better picture of my long-term prognosis.

Well, in the course of an hour-and-a-half visit, the neurologist concluded that I had "extremely diminished strength in my right arm and hand." *Duh!* I could've told him that at the *start* of the appointment!! (Just as an aside, when I received the bill for this neurologist's ninety-minute "consultation," the tab was $1,642! My health insurance paid a whopping 49 bucks! Guess who paid the rest? *Moi!*) Oh, also, the neurologist wanted me to see a "spinal specialist." When I asked why, he replied, "In case you end up in the emergency room, there will be a doctor who would know your history."

During this entire six-month ordeal, my sister pleaded with me to talk to her mother-in-law who worked for a family chiropractor. Finally, I called my sister's mother-in-law, and proceeded to spill my tale of woe and how the medical doctors were pushing me to have surgery! She immediately told me to STOP! She said she hadn't seen a medical doctor in 30 years. This God-sent mother-in-law-of-my-sister began to tell me about the advantages of Chiropractic care and how everything comes from the spine.

The next day, she referred me to three chiropractors in my area posted in an online nationwide directory. I selected Dr. DeMoss from the list and the rest is history! It's a *miracle*—no kidding!! And I mean this with all sincerity! At first, I was a "What have I got to lose?" skeptic. I was already pretty-much resigned to neck surgery as a desperate measure to stop the unbearable pain. After all, when a medical specialist tells you that you need surgery, you tend to believe them! Right? *Not so fast!*

Well, I've been seeing Dr. DeMoss for two-and-a-half months. I'm no longer taking *any* medication, and I haven't since a week after my first visit. I also have no more pain...the numbness in my arm and hand has diminished to the point that I don't even notice it. I'm able to sleep on my right side through the entire night. Sheer Bliss! And the best part of all: I'm able to work out, run, ride horses, go boating, and...yes...*ski!* Everything!

Just before I met Dr. DeMoss, I couldn't work out or do *any* kind of physical activity.... It was horrible. I remember on my last trip to the orthopedist for Novocain-and-cortisone shots and more pain medication, my husband asked what he could do to help me. All I said was, "I just want my life back!" And I burst into tears. You don't realize how important good health is until you don't have it any longer! Dr. DeMoss has given me my life back and saved me from surgery. And you know what? None of those medical doctors could do that for me!

I've also learned from Dr. DeMoss how over-medicated our society is. Big Pharma Rules! Think about it: We tend to look to medical doctors for *everything*, and all I see them doing is prescribing and over-prescribing medication and surgery. These remedies are probably good for *something*; but at this point, I'm not at all sure what!

I've got my life back...and I thank Dr. DeMoss for that!

Lori Dahl
Chiropractic advocate and
Grateful patient of
Billy DeMoss, DC
DeMoss Chiropractic
Newport Beach, California

The Boy Who Touched My Heart

Kevin was a remarkable young man whose parents brought him from Belgium to America in search of healing. Born with a debilitating condition—cerebral palsy, Kevin suffered all his life as he fought to overcome its crippling effects. The disease rendered him unable to walk, stand, or sit up straight without assistance.

As a boy of thirteen—bound to a wheelchair—Kevin had been forced to cope with numerous challenges every single day. His loving parents sought therapy for their son from medical doctors and healers too numerous to count! Just one of the well-intentioned treatments involved actually cutting contracted muscles in his legs in order to release tension. The numerous scars on Kevin's legs give quiet testimony to these failed "cures" administered with a surgeon's scalpel.

The parents' quest to improve the quality of Kevin's life brought them to America for intensive physical therapy with a world-renowned physician to help their boy learn how to walk. I found out about Kevin and his family while they were guests of an American family who were patients of mine. In turn, the American family told them about the Chiropractic care from which they had benefitted. At first, Kevin's parents were apprehensive, tired of disappointing results they had experienced at the hands of well-meaning medical doctors. On the other hand, they were willing to explore every avenue for the sake of their son. After careful thought, they finally decided to give Chiropractic a try.

I remember the day I met Kevin and his parents; and I knew what they were thinking: "After all the healthcare experts we've seen, what could a *chiropractor* possibly accomplish for our son?" I knew that God had brought Kevin to my office for a reason; and I felt an immediate, loving bond with him. I examined the boy thoroughly and committed in my heart that I would do everything possible to help this child as if he were my own.

The challenges Kevin faced were many. He always sat in a slumped position due to muscle weakness in his spine. He couldn't turn himself over on the adjusting table without help from his parents. Having no flexibility in his feet, he had extreme difficulty walking up and down stairs, and could not walk at all without the use of braces and crutches. He even wore leg braces to bed so his muscles would not contract while he slept. His energy level was low, and he required a lot of rest. Kevin's handwriting was comparable to that of a kindergarten-age child, and he needed constant assistance for most of his daily tasks.

The day after Kevin's Chiropractic assessment, he came in for his first adjustment. The night before, I prayed to God that a miracle would be created in Kevin's life. Now, here was the moment of truth. While I worked on Kevin, he kept repeating "Dr. Maloof [that's me] is a Genie." After I finished his first adjustment, he sat up straight—without assistance—for the first time in his life. His huge smile and enormous energy lit up the entire office! Kevin was a changed person—as if "the lights had been turned on in his body." Even patients in the waiting room commented on the aura of energy and light surrounding him. Kevin politely kissed my hands and said to his parents, "I *told* you she was a Genie." I felt totally connected with Kevin and was thrilled that God had begun to answer my prayers. Kevin's physical therapist—and everyone else—noticed incredible improvements after the first Chiropractic adjustment.

Kevin came in the next day and his parents were very excited, telling me how much more energetic and happy their son had become. In the following days—after each adjustment—Kevin showered me with hugs and kisses of gratitude.

After the third adjustment, I told Kevin to go home and write a letter. He complained, saying he couldn't write well. I insisted! He came in the next day with a perfectly handwritten letter that shocked everyone. He subsequently mailed it to his grandmother. She later asked, "Who wrote the letter for you?" Grandma couldn't believe Kevin had written it himself.

Kevin's treatment consisted of Chiropractic adjustments to correct vertebral subluxations—misaligned vertebrae pinching nerves—resulting from birth trauma. By removing nerve interference, the function of his muscles was greatly enhanced. In turn, this made possible improved flexibility and posture. I employed many different techniques to adjust his spine, cranium, temporomandibular joint (TMJ) or jaw hinge, elbows, wrists, legs, and feet. I also tested him for nutritional deficiencies and gave him supplements to help strengthen his muscles.

After Kevin's sixth adjustment, my heart was filled with joy and hope as he walked down the office hallway *without braces for the first time in his life.* That day, Kevin was wearing a tee shirt featuring then-basketball star Dennis Rodman's picture and the boy told me Rodman was his hero. As if Kevin's walking that day were not a big enough miracle, I met Dennis Rodman that very evening at a Laker's game and was able to share Kevin's story with the star. Rodman then autographed a tee shirt for Kevin. I was so excited, I barely slept that night; I couldn't wait to tell Kevin the story! Needless to say, when Kevin heard about my encounter the previous evening and was given the autographed shirt, he was ecstatic!!

Finally, there was only one week left before Kevin had to return to Belgium. I did my best to make optimal use of the precious time remaining. Encouraging me on, his mother regularly commented, "Kevin would walk *slowly* and *carefully* into the doctor's office and—after his adjustment—he would practically *run* out the door." The grip strength in Kevin's hands improved by 20 pounds after only ten adjustments, and his leg strength went from zero to full scale. He was able to turn himself over on the table without assistance and even climbed into the van by himself. He was able to walk up and down stairs with ease and no longer slept with leg braces. His feet became flexible, and he could walk without braces or crutches.

The most difficult part of the treatment came when we had to say goodbye. Kevin's ever-present love—and a new smile that could brighten any room—made him a joy to be around. Our farewell was filled with hugs, kisses, tears, and heartache. I felt as if I was saying goodbye to my own son. With God's help, Chiropractic had restored Kevin's health, and Kevin's healing touched my heart.

Catherine Maloof, DC
Maloof Chiropractic
Mission Viejo, California

Dr. Maloof is the author of
Healthy Eating One Bite at a Time
and
Renew Your Heart One Beat at a Time

Scary Story with a Happy Ending

"I believe that you can, by taking some simple and inexpensive measures, extend your life and your years of well-being. My most important recommendation is that you take vitamins every day, in optimum amounts, to supplement the vitamins you receive in your food."

Linus Pauling, PhD
Two-time Nobel Laureate: Chemistry and Peace
(1901-1994)

I was scared—and had good reason to be! I was suffering with pneumonia and had severe difficulty breathing. My medical doctors diagnosed the problem as a "loculated pleural effusion"—a fibrotic mass. The mass I was hosting occupied 35 percent of my left lung!

My search for relief took me to the world-famous Cleveland Clinic where the top surgeons told me I needed a "thoracotomy" to remove the mass from my lung. When they explained what that entailed, I got REALLY scared. With the proposed procedure, I'd be subjected to a general anesthesia. Then, a heart-lung machine would take over those vital functions while the surgeons temporarily "disconnected" some of the ribs attached to my spine to allow access to the affected lung! Furthermore, they offered no guarantee that this risky procedure would resolve my breathing problems! Wouldn't *you* be scared? I WANTED A SECOND OPINION!

In my forty-year career as a chiropractor, I've made the acquaintance of a large number of wonderful, talented people including a brilliant cardiologist who embraces the fact that proper nutrition, daily exercise, and regular Chiropractic mainte-nance can do wonders in sustaining health and wellness. When I called him for a second-opinion referral, he arranged an appoint-ment for me with the head of thoracic surgery at the world-famous Brigham and Women's Hospital in Boston, a teaching affiliate of the Harvard Medical School.

After a thorough workup, the Boston specialists agreed with their colleagues at the Cleveland Clinic—I needed a thoracotomy or *I would soon die of pneumonia!* I was told to go home and rest up so I could get in the best possible shape—considering my circumstances—to better withstand, and recover from, the surgery. From a scheduling standpoint, I would be in the hospital for two weeks following the operation plus another four-to-five months at home for recovery. Since Christmas was approaching, I decided to postpone my surgery until after the New Year rather than subject my family to any sort of holiday vigil.

Now, this mass in my lung didn't simply come from nowhere; so let me tell you how my medical nightmare began. Two years ago, when I was 63, I started having mild chest pain. I hoped that, if I just ignored it, this inconvenient nuisance would just behave itself and go away. After about six months of denial, and with my wife's encouragement, I got an exam.

The medical doctors told me I had some sort of "coronary insufficiency," but they weren't sure exactly what it was. More test-ing revealed that my cholesterol was fine! My blood pressure was fine! My weight and "body-mass-index" were fine! A CT scan of my chest revealed nothing conclusive. But the pain persisted.

Then, a coronary specialist suggested a series of diagnostics including a thallium stress test. I was injected intravenously with a mildly-radioactive thallium solution and then got on a treadmill. It took ten minutes at full speed before my heart rate got up to the required level—I was in *great* shape. Then, I lay down on my back and a special camera photographed my heart to determine how the various chambers had filled up with thallium. (On the resulting image, a "glowing" chamber is getting all the blood it needs; a "not-so-bright" chamber is suffering some sort of blockage.)

The test revealed that my coronary insufficiency was in the left ventricle—in particular, the *left anterior descending* artery emerging from the left ventricle. This "LAD"—also known as the "widow maker" since its complete blockage will, without exception, result in a fatal heart attack with no possibility of recovery—had an anomalous ninety-degree kink in it! Apparently, I had had this problem since birth! The doctors told me that, if I had not been in such good health—if I had been a big drinker or a heavy smoker, I would probably have died in my fifties!

The next step was installation of a "stent" to eliminate potential further blockage of the LAD. To do this, a "cardiac catheterization" was called for in which a collapsed metal-mesh tube is inserted through an artery in the groin, threaded up into the LAD next to the heart, and then expanded. Unfortunately, in my case, it was discovered *during the procedure* that the angle in my LAD was so extreme that expansion of the stent could rupture the artery. Not good! The procedure was aborted. But the potential *widow maker* was still lurking, waiting to wreak havoc!

Next step: Bypass Surgery! Under general anesthesia, with heart-lung machine support, my ribs were opened up using a "chest spreader" to provide access to my LAD. Then, they harvested my mammary artery and used it to bypass the LAD. Finally, the surgical team closed me up again.

Following surgery, I continued my regular regimen of daily exercise and whole food supplements plus weekly adjustments. Six months later, though, while playing a round of golf, I got really tired and very weak. I found out in the emergency room that I had contracted pneumonia; and the doctor ordered a CAT scan. That's when they discovered the accumulation of blood seepage on the inside of chest—in the "pleura" or sac the lungs fit into—

due to a complication resulting from the surgery. The doctor explained that while the seepage was tiny, "Sooner or later, a dripping faucet can fill a bathtub."

I spent the next five months trying to recover with natural methods. Then, I got pneumonia a second time. I couldn't walk more than 50 steps. I lost my ability to breathe. In search of relief, I went to the Cleveland Clinic—where this story began. But that's NOT where this story ends!

You'll remember that I decided to build up my strength and spend the Christmas holidays with my family before my thoracotomy under the scalpel of a world-famous surgeon at the Brigham and Women's Hospital in Boston. Given the risk posed by this operation, I wanted to spend time with Donna, my wife of 44 years; Jim, my oldest son—a fellow chiropractor, and his wife, Christine; Bob, my second son—a naturopath, and his wife, Beth; my daughter Heather and her husband, Chip Null, who is a second-career chiropractor; my daughter Andrea and her husband, Dan Smith, who is another second-career chiropractor; and my thirteen grandchildren!

By the time the New Year rolled around, I had enjoyed a few months of rest, mild exercise, daily whole food supplements, and weekly adjustments administered by my oldest son. Quite simply, I was feeling pretty darn good! My cardiologist suggested that I get another CAT scan before scheduling surgery. That's what I did! Come to find out, the mass had resolved itself down to less than 10 percent where the previous scan had registered 35 percent! I went back to the thoracic surgeon; he said there was no reason to operate. Somehow or other, my body had reabsorbed most of that mass—a rare phenomenon according to the surgeon, since the mass is a fibrous material.

My wife and I burst into tears of relief. The miracle of it is that I had people praying for me all over the country. I also believe that with natural methods, if you give the body enough time to heal, it sometimes can heal the most difficult maladies.

Luckily, I waited long enough. If I had just jumped into the surgery, I'd still be recovering—with no long-term guarantees!

Bear in mind, I'm not yet 100 percent! I'm still a little short of breath, and I don't have the lung capacity that I had prior to the heart surgery. But I'm so grateful that I don't take *any* medication. My wife and I walk a mile together every morning. AND I'm working full time! Our family operates a large Chiropractic clinic with four skilled doctors and a naturopath on staff. I'm also privileged to serve as a consultant to Standard Process, a Palmyra, Wisconsin-based manufacturer of whole food dietary supplements—a key part of the nutrition regimen that helped me recover from my lung disorder.

It is the belief system of every chiropractor that the body has—within it—the ability to heal itself. And since God created the human body, I give God the credit for its beautiful design. By His grace, I'm still here.

James P. Powell, DC
Powell Chiropractic Clinic
Canton, Ohio

Consultant to
Standard Process Inc.
Whole Food Supplements Since 1929

As told to Don Dible

11

Chiropractic and Sports

"The team wasn't just riders. It was the mechanics, masseurs, chefs, soigneurs, and doctors. But the most important man on the team may have been the chiropractor."
Lance Armstrong, 7 time Tour de France Champion

"… as long as I see the chiropractor,
I feel like I`m one step ahead of the game."
Tom Brady, Quarterback, New England Patriots
3 time Superbowl Champion and 2 time Superbowl MVP

"Without Chiropractic, I wouldn't be able
to play consistently throughout the season."
Johnny Damon, Centerfielder, New York Yankees
World Series Champion with the Boston Red Sox

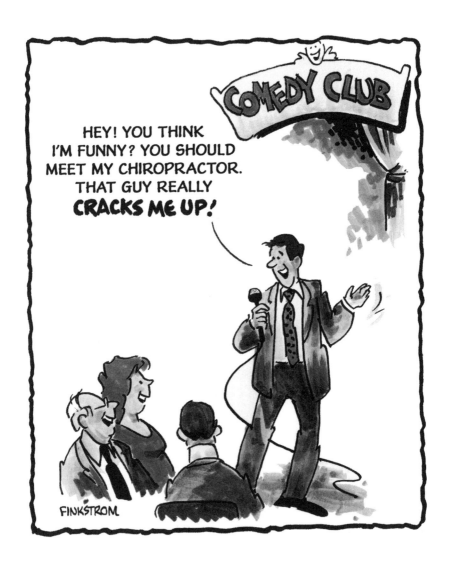

Teddi's New "Favorite Thing to Do"

Teddi was five-years old when she had her first seizure—just three weeks after we were involved in a car accident. Her neurologist didn't link the accident with the onset of her seizures even though, prior to the accident, she had never had an episode. This was the beginning of a very rough road for my little girl.

Each episode wiped out Teddi's memory, causing her to fall further and further behind in school. To make matters worse, these seizures would often completely paralyze her right side—symptoms often experienced by stroke victims. Sadly, the doctors weren't much help. Each time she had a seizure, they would increase her medication levels—leaving her with even more challenges. The medicines sedated her so much that she couldn't function normally in a classroom. Some of the drugs precipitated anti-social behavior, making her very difficult to manage at home *and* at school. In the beginning, I was hopeful that this disorder—like many other challenges in life—was something Teddi would simply outgrow. As the years passed, however, my hope of her ever getting her life back faded. Although I couldn't give up, I didn't know how else to help her. In fact, I felt help-*less!*

Epilepsy quickly took over all of our lives including those of Teddi's brother and sister. They were affected due to the limitations on things our family could do or places we could go. We simply were unable to predict when her next random seizure might occur. Teddi's siblings couldn't understand why such a beautiful, happy, loving, sweet girl had to deal with this horrible disorder. I couldn't satisfactorily explain to them why this was happening. They spent countless weekends in training classes and sibling support groups to help them cope with a sister afflicted with this horrible disorder.

After struggling for more than five years—and fed up with feeling helpless, I enrolled in an anatomy and physiology continuing education course in the hope of learning more about my daughter's disability. The instructor—an intern at the Parker College of Chiropractic in Dallas—was only too happy to answer a few after-class questions regarding the nervous system. When I gave him some basic information about Teddi, he shared her story with Dr. Carrie Ann Gallagher, a pediatric specialist intern also at Parker. Carrie Ann quickly took Teddi under her wing and brought her in for an evaluation including head, neck, and spinal x-rays plus a comprehensive physical exam and thermal and EMG scans of her back. She found that Teddi had many spinal subluxations.

When Teddi began Chiropractic treatment at the age of nine, she was on extremely high dosages of anti-convulsive medication that severely affected her quality of life. She was still having seizures on an almost-daily basis. After just sixteen Chiropractic visits—spanning a period of five weeks, we were able to start decreasing Teddi's medications and still go for weeks without a seizure. After Teddi had received five months of Chiropractic care, her neurologist insisted that we didn't have her on enough medications to control her seizures. During that same five-month period, Teddi had experienced only three seizures. Ignoring the advice of her neurologist, we continued to decrease Teddi's medication, changed her diet, and made Chiropractic care an integral part of her everyday life.

One year before starting treatment with Carrie Ann, Teddi wasn't able to swim, go to a friend's birthday party, or even have dinner in a restaurant without risking a seizure. She celebrated her tenth birthday at a local indoor pool where she played with her friends and swam. Teddi's new "favorite thing to do" is jumping off the diving board—just like her brother and sister. I can't begin to tell you what this has meant for Teddi and our whole family. Thanks to Chiropractic, epilepsy isn't controlling our lives any more.

Sandi Rosier, LMT, MTI
Mother of Teddi Rosier

Teddi's adjustments were performed by
Carrie Ann Gallagher, DC, at
Parker College of Chiropractic
Dallas, Texas

Dr. Gallagher is now seeing patients at
Beingwell Healthcare
Prahran, Victoria
AUSTRALIA

Adapted from an article appearing in
Pathways to Family Wellness magazine
Published by the
International Chiropractic Pediatric Association, Inc.

One-Hundred and Twenty-Six Days

At the age of fifteen, I was injured in a football game. That event radically changed my life.

I still remember the exact day on which I got hurt and the minute, blow-by-blow details leading up to my injury. I was a freshman at Livingston High School and played fullback on the football team. My mother didn't want me to play because she was afraid I'd get hurt and not be able to play baseball. While baseball has always been my first love, I felt like football was something I just had to try or else I'd never know if it was right for me. Well, I found out the hard way that it was not!

On a chilly, windy day in late September, we played our first scrimmage. That game was also my last. In the first play, I received a handoff and made a mad dash for the end zone. I successfully evaded broken and missed tackles until the only thing separating me from a touchdown was one man. As the distance between us closed, I faked left and went right. He dove and grabbed my leg as my fake was in process. At the same time, a middle linebacker was pursuing me hard from behind and hit my lower spine with his helmet. At the point of impact, I fell instantly and couldn't move. I lay on the ground for what seemed like an eternity. A million thoughts rushed through my head as the trainers hesitated to move me because of my pain. After lying there for some time, all my thoughts started to drift off except one: "Was I ever going to play baseball again?"

I was out for the rest of the football season and tried to rest up for baseball. The trainer worked on me all the way up to the spring trying to rehabilitate my injury. The spring came and I played baseball. I wasn't even close to a hundred percent; but not playing would have hurt even more than the physical pain I was feeling. The pain continued through the summer and fall baseball season. At the end of the fall, during one of the games, I got a base hit and started to run. Suddenly, I realized something was wrong. The feeling in my legs was gone and the pain in my back was excruciating.

After the game, I told my mom, and she took me to a nearby orthopedic doctor. The pain that I had blocked out for so long had increased to the point I couldn't block it anymore. This had never happened to me before. My tolerance for pain is normally very high; that's how I knew something was definitely wrong this time. After the orthopedist made some tests, he sat my mom and me down and told us he didn't think I was ever going to be able to play *any* physical sport again. He said I had damaged my lower spine so badly it would be nearly impossible for me to continue.

As I sat there, tears started rolling down my cheeks; it was like a part of me was gone. After that, I promised myself I wouldn't go to any more doctors and just continue to tough it out until I dropped. I've never trusted doctors in the first place because I always feared they'd say I couldn't play. Now, this fear came true; and I'd have to rely on a determined heart to carry me through the pain.

Although this approach worked for a while, the pain kept getting worse and worse. One night, a friend of my mom came over for dinner and recommended that I go see Dr. Donna. She said she was sure she could help. Well, my first reaction was, "No way am I going to another doctor!"

She told me that Dr. Donna was a chiropractor; and if she couldn't help me she'd come straight out and say it. After a lot of arguing, I went to see her. At my first visit, she didn't waste any time. Dr. Donna immediately sent me for an MRI to see what was going on.

Based on the resulting images, Dr. Donna found that I had two herniated disks *and* two bulging disks. Without hesitation, I asked her if she could fix me so I could play pain-free again. She said she felt she could, but "It will take time."

Time was something I didn't have too much of. I sat on the table and said, "I've never trusted doctors in my life, but if you get me in good enough shape to play in one-hundred-and-twenty-six days, I'll trust you." That was the amount of time that remained until the start of baseball season.

She looked me straight in the eyes and, with a caring, warm, and confident stare replied, "Let's go to work!"

Those one-hundred-and-twenty-six days were days I'll never forget. By the end, I was able to do things that I never thought I'd be able to do again. Why is this? It's because Dr. Donna and her staff cared about me. There are many words that describe Dr. Donna: "Caring," "Kind," "Loving," "Determined," and "Confident." My favorite word to describe her is "Best" because she is the "BEST." If it wasn't for her, my body would have eventually given up; and I would have never been able to play again. I'm now in college and still playing the one sport I truly love.

I frequently think about the challenges I gave Dr. Donna that day in her examining room. I now go to her with all of my college baseball injuries. She's helped me heal sprained ankles, wrist problems, torn cartilage in my fingers, disk problems, and is currently adjusting my ribs since I'm having bad chest pains. There's nothing this lady cannot do; I trust her with my *life!* I don't know how to repay her for all she has done and the patience she has shown me. For now, all I can say is, "Thank you, Dr. Donna, from the bottom of my heart."

Thomas L. Kroeger II
Thankful patient of
Donna Cantalupo, DC
Chiropractic Center of East Hanover
East Hanover, New Jersey

Beijing 2008 and the Well-Adjusted Team

"Were it not for Chiropractic, I would not have won the gold medal!"

Dan O'Brien—Double Olympic and World
Championship Decathlon Gold Medalist

This is a story about Chiropractic and the winning of a Silver Medal by the U.S. Olympic Men's Water Polo Team at the Beijing Summer Olympics in 2008—the *first* U.S. medal in that event since our team won a Silver Medal at the Seoul Summer Olympics 20 years earlier! But before I can tell this story, I need to gently put modesty aside and fill you in on the influence of Chiropractic in my life and the road to my becoming official chiropractor and head coach of the U.S. Olympic Men's Water Polo Team.

Starting with my paternal grandfather, there is a lineage of 69 chiropractors—male and female—in our family! My understanding is that *ours is the largest Chiropractic family in the world.* Like his father, my dad became a chiropractor; and dad set up his office in our home. Chiropractic was the primary family health-care practiced there. (I've never taken an aspirin; I've never been vaccinated.) As children aged nine and ten, my brother, Lance, and I—both delivered by my father—were fascinated as we regularly observed people enter our father's office with the aid of one or two canes, crutches, or, in some cases, carried in. (When she got a little older, our much-younger sister, Tammy, was able to observe the same phenomena.) Then, the office door would close and our father would do whatever it is that chiropractors do. In fifteen to twenty minutes, the door would open again and many of those patients would walk out under their own power while joking, laughing, and smiling. My brother and I concluded that our dad was a miracle man! He helped lots of people, and we decided we also wanted to help people by doing whatever it was that he did—we committed ourselves to becoming *chiropractors!* Not surprisingly, our sister later made the same career choice. I received my Doctor of Chiropractic degree in 1986.

As a freshman at Pepperdine University in 1976, I made the water polo team where I played for four seasons. This led to my selection to the USA National team from which I was subsequently named to the 1980 Olympic team—the first of four Olympic Games in which I participated as a member of the USA water polo team. Chiropractic played a huge role in helping me to become the only four-time Olympian in the sport of water polo in America. I had served as head coach of the Pepperdine Waves men's water polo team from 1986 to 2005. (We actually won a national championship in 1997.) In 2007, USA Water Polo asked me to become the head coach of our 2008 Olympic team.

I looked at this opportunity from a couple of different perspectives. One was the obvious honor of being an Olympic head coach. But, just as important to me was the honor and privilege of bringing Chiropractic to a deeper level for this team. I already knew many of the members, having coached them—or observed them as members of opposing teams in the college ranks—during my 20-years as head coach at Pepperdine.

We started full-time training for the Olympics in early 2007 at the California Lutheran University and the Oaks Christian High School, both in Thousand Oaks, California. Most of my Pepperdine players had already been exposed to Chiropractic as had many of the players from the other teams. I was regularly able to adjust a lot of the guys and was assisted by our trainer-strength coach, Eric Goodman, an intern at the Los Angeles College of Chiropractic. It was kind of fun to see some of the guys that I had previously worked on when I was coaching. They already knew that the benefit of Chiropractic was way beyond simple pain relief. They understood, as athletes, that Chiropractic care could actually help them with their performance by keeping their spines in alignment and their finely-tuned nervous systems functioning at the highest possible level.

As we went through that year-and-a-half run up to Beijing, more and more of our athletes observed the benefits of Chiropractic for their teammates and also wanted that perform-ance-enhancing edge. Among the more vocal advocates was Merrill Moses, our goalie, who continually talked about how good he felt and how the adjustments were helping him. Before we left for Beijing, a handful of our athletes were still fearful and didn't want anything to do with Chiropractic. They couldn't even watch teammates being adjusted; they were especially afraid of having their necks manipulated. Some would even turn their backs rather than watch the procedure.

After a while, one of our big centers, six-foot-six-inch Ryan Bailey, came over to me and said, "Coach, I'm afraid of being adjusted, but my neck is *killing* me. Can you please check it out and give me an adjustment? Just be gentle." After that first adjustment, he was really pleased and excited. While he didn't get adjusted as often as Merrill, he had discovered the benefits and got adjusted on a more regular basis. Still another athlete, Peter Varellas, who played one of our "attacker" positions, ultimately became open to Chiropractic.

After almost a year of preparation in Thousand Oaks, we traveled to Belgrade in February 2008 to train with the Serbian team. The first night after our arrival, we scrimmaged with them and got hammered 17-3! We were in Belgrade for ten days and scrimmaged every day. Our last scrimmage was an "official game" in which we were beaten 14-6. What made the loss all the more humiliating is that half the Serbian team came to the game straight from Happy Hour! On the trip home, we clearly had our tails between our legs and realized we had a heck of a lot of work to do before Beijing!

In May, the reigning world water polo champions from Croatia visited our Thousand Oaks facility to train and engage us in a couple of scrimmages. We lost the first game, but the margin was respectable. In the second game, we beat the Croats 7-5. At that point, you could see the U.S. team mindset begin to shift; you could feel our confidence start to build—the sea-change in attitude was palpable! *There was a growing realization that we had a fighting chance to medal in Beijing!*

In June, we traveled to Cosenza, Italy, for the FINA [Federation Internationale de Natation] Water Polo World League Tournament in which the world's top eight teams compete. We made it to the finals against Serbia. At the end of the third quarter, the score was tied. Although we ultimately lost the game, we recognized that we had given the Serbs a run for their money. We had improved so much in just four months that our confidence reached new highs.

When we arrived at the Olympic Games, the U.S. men's team was ranked ninth in the world. We beat China in our first game. Next, we upset Italy and moved on to conquer Croatia. Germany fell to our onslaught before we moved into the semi-finals to face our old nemesis, Serbia. Looking back, that was a *beautiful* game: we won by a compelling score of 10-5! That was a HUGE turnaround from where we had been in February, and the U.S. team was *guaranteed* a place on the medal podium!

Two days after our victory over Serbia, we entered the Olympic final where we faced Hungary—a formidable adversary. Our defense, which had only allowed six goals per game going into the final, became a little porous. At the half, we were down 9-8, and felt as though we'd already played an entire game. The

Hungarians were shooting the ball extremely well and discovering holes in our defense.

Hungary had won the Sydney Summer Olympics Men's Water Polo Gold Medal in 2000. Hungary had won the Los Angeles Summer Olympics Men's Water Polo Gold Medal in 2004. And Hungary won the Beijing Summer Olympics Men's Water Polo Gold Medal in 2008 with a score of 14-9! Our team had to be content with the Silver Medal—the first medal of any kind won by a U.S. men's team in this sport in two decades! Obviously, that brought back a lot of pride in U.S. men's water polo.

I had the opportunity to watch the Bronze Medal game between Serbia and Montenegro. When I saw the joy and celebration of the Serbs after they won that game, I was fascinated by the contrast in seeing the bittersweet reaction of our team after we lost to Hungary and won the silver. We had a lot to be proud of. Nine of the thirteen guys on our 2008 Olympic team are now training and working for the 2012 Games in the hope of winning that Gold Medal in London. And I'm still coaching them!

Merrill Moses, our vocal goalie, is now among those training for the 2012 Games. He's also taking the undergraduate prerequisites for his study to become a Doctor of Chiropractic!

Just as the U.S. Olympic Men's Water Polo Team has come a long way, so too has the 47-member 2010 U.S. Olympic Committee Medical Staff whose new Director is Dr. Michael Reed—a Chiropractor!

Terry A. Schroeder, DC
Schroeder Center for Healthy Living
Westlake Village, California
As told to Don Dible

Passion for Speed!

"I envy them for being so at home in the wild world,
wide open to its beauty, plugged into its power. For
whatever it is they find there that proves so irresistible."

Author Maria Coffey—whose soulmate perished while
ascending Mt. Everest—discussing big mountain
snowboarders and climbers in her book,
Explorers of the Infinite

June 25, 2000, marked the end of my "first life"...as a speed-obsessed, eighteen-year-old athlete in peak physical condition—and the start of a new one...as a medically-diagnosed quadriplegic. This is my story.

When I was one-year old—before I could walk—my mother, Kay Ledson, put me on the seat of a tiny BMX bike. I quickly dropped the training wheels! She put me on skis when I was two. I quickly got rid of the poles! I started snowboarding at eleven and competed internationally at fifteen. What drives me? *Speed is FREEDOM!*

In 1998, I spent four months in Switzerland as an exchange student. Every chance I got, I'd hone my snowboarding skills—especially long aerial jumps—in the nearby Swiss Alps. One day, while attempting a particularly long jump, I landed on my back and broke a lumbar vertebra. It wasn't until I returned home to Australia that the fracture was diagnosed and I came into the rehabilitative care of a brilliant chiropractor, Dr. Simon Floreani. Over the next two years, Simon prescribed a regimen of gentle spinal adjustments, proper diet, nutritional supplements, and carefully-monitored exercise.

On June 23, 2000, during a routine office visit, Simon told me I was completely rehabilitated. That was GREAT news since I had just secured lodging accommodations and a season pass at the Mt. Buller Ski Resort a few hours' drive northeast of Melbourne. I planned to secure employment at Buller and practice snowboarding at every opportunity in order to become a professional.

On Saturday, June 24th, a bunch of my mates left their BMX and motocross bikes at home, loaded up their snowboards, and joined me at Buller. Since I had recently returned from another snowboard-jumping visit to Switzerland, I was eager to duplicate my Swiss acrobatics on home turf. The problem was that Buller had no comparable long-distance jumps.

Saturday night, we discussed the fact that nobody had yet jumped a two-year-old, 75-foot-wide access road that cut across a closed ski/snowboard trail. Sunday morning, we found the perfect spot to build a pair of jump-the-road ramps. Soon after we started, a member of the Mt. Buller Ski Patrol stopped by, discussed our plans, and provided preliminary approval. To gather material for the site, my mates and I rolled snowman-sized "snowballs" down the mountain. To make the launch ramp slippery, we sprinkled a bit of salt to ice the surface. After five hours' work, we finished and the Ski Patrol gave us a final okay.

Since I had the most experience, my friends decided I should go first. Accompanied by my two best mates, I climbed high enough on the trail to attain maximum velocity at the launch ramp; mounted my board; and waited for a signal from my friends below that no vehicles were approaching. Then, with a best mate on my left and right, they grabbed my hands and flung me—like the projectile from a slingshot—straight down the fall line.

In seconds, I hit the icy launch ramp and was airborne.

Moments later, I was upside-down!

The curve on the ramp proved just a bit too sharp; I was going just a bit too fast. And my knees buckled...just a bit... *critically cutting my speed!* Reflexively, my feet pushed away from my hips, thus initiating a rotation that flipped me 180 degrees. In midair, I realized I wasn't going to make it to the other ramp…my too-high trajectory was about seven feet short of the required 75 feet—and peaked about sixteen feet above the asphalt. Just before I hit the road, I tucked my head in—so I wouldn't crush my skull or get a concussion—and attempted an army-style forward roll.

On impact, my chin got buried in my chest. When I bounced off the road, my head whiplashed back and my helmet hit between my shoulder blades. I heard a massive BANG—like the discharge of a shotgun at close range. Straightaway, I knew my neck was broken!

"I've broken my neck, don't touch me!" I shouted at my friends as they rushed to my aid. Twisted like a pretzel, I thought my spine had actually come through my chest.

I asked one of my friends to confirm this, and he said, "Josh, nothing's there."

Everything was like hot rushes. I had no feeling in my hands or legs. "Can you get that rock out from under my back?" I asked.

"Josh, nothing's there."

My mates packed snow around my shoulders and hips to stabilize me. One held onto my head—which felt like it wasn't attached to my body. Stoked with adrenaline, I kept joking until I started slipping in and out of consciousness. I became very relaxed…then floppy. Next, I stiffened up before starting mild convulsions. I swallowed my tongue; and my mate pulled it out of my airway to stop me from choking.

After the Mt. Buller Medical Centre team arrived, they carefully removed my board and boots and cut away my jacket. I was rushed to the medical facility for x-rays and an MRI. Everything confirmed what I already knew: my neck was broken. Steroids were injected into my spinal cord to reduce swelling.

Once stabilized, I was airlifted to the Austin Hospital—the prominent spinal-injury facility in Melbourne—where my parents waited anxiously. I don't remember much about the following week because I was drugged to the eyeballs. My parents were told I was a C-5, C-6, C-7, T-1 complete quadriplegic. C-7, the seventh cervical vertebra counting down from my head, was completely destroyed when I slammed into the asphalt. My prognosis was dire. If I survived, it was unlikely I'd ever get out of bed since my spinal cord was badly crushed. Like my neck, my mother's heart broke.

Four days later, the Austin Hospital surgeon made an incision alongside my throat. Working through that opening, he removed practically my entire C-7 vertebra—in tiny bits-and-pieces—and replaced it with bone "harvested" from my hips to provide a protective barrier around my spinal cord. To stabilize my spine, a titanium plate was attached with screws to the front of C-6 and T-1, the vertebrae above and below my now-useless C-7. The three vertebrae were thus fused like a single block of bone to provide a protective barrier around the spinal cord and prevent it from being further compressed or tethered.

While I was in a morphine-induced stupor Sunday night, my mum asked the hospital staff if my chiropractor could see me since he was extremely familiar with my nervous system. They flatly refused.

Now one of Mum's many endearing characteristics is that she's occasionally "selectively deaf." This was one of those times. At 6:30am on the day after my accident, she arrived at Simon's practice and explained what had happened. He visited me at the Austin Hospital that evening posing as my "snowboarding coach." With very, very gentle and specific adjustments and rehab techniques, he immediately set about helping to keep my spinal cord alive. He later explained that tradi-tional management leaves these injuries with swelling and inflammation around the spinal cord—shutting down the flow of intelligence between the brain and the rest of the body. The brain's signals get traffic-jammed at the injury site...permanently.

Simon's thinking was, "If we steadily and safely remind Josh's brain that it needs to keep logged in and connected to the rest of his body, we can avoid the usual nerve atrophy that results when painkillers shut *everything* down." It wasn't long after that when I pressed my doctors to radically reduce the quantity of painkillers and other drugs I was on. Almost immediately, my brain started reconnecting with my body despite MRI evidence showing less than ten percent spinal cord function.

Simon later explained that our hands and feet have the highest representation on the surface of the brain. In order to keep my brain interacting with my extremities, he adjusted my fingers and toes every day. He also gave instructions to Mum that all of my friends should stop crying when they visited and, instead, massage my fingers and toes. Mum also brought in a dear family friend, Rose, who joined my rehab team and taught me visualization and how to use the intense pain to guide me.

As I look back on my early recovery, I had a number of fascinating mind-body experiences. For example, I'd be lying in bed with my arms at my sides and my legs dead straight while my brain was telling me my left foot was resting behind my head and that my arms were all twisted. While *some* intelligence was getting to my brain, that intelligence was *confusing!*

With Simon's help, I started working through a lot of visualization. What was most effective was imagining that I had a video camera scanning my body. Since I knew my arms and legs were straight, I'd mentally send the "video camera" to those locations and override the confusing messages. After about a week of mind-numbing concentration, it started to work! Before long, I was able to wiggle the big toe on my left foot. You can't possibly imagine how exciting that simple achievement was for me.

Mum also pitched in. One day shortly after I entered the hospital, a surgeon at my bedside was explaining very carefully—and with condescending certainty—that I needed a "reality check." "Y-o-u...a-r-e...a...q-u-a-d-r-i-p-l-e-g-i-c; you will *never* snowboard or ride a motorbike again; you're going to spend *the rest of your life* in a wheelchair!

Mum overheard him and shouted: "Doctor, we are *positive people!* If you don't have anything *positive* to say, then say *absolutely nothing!* Do I make myself clear?"

Relentlessly searching for *any* positive input, Mum sent my MRIs to close family friends in California. They forwarded them to a renowned spinal surgeon at Cedars-Sinai Medical Center in Los Angeles. His prognosis: *Josh will never walk again!"*

Incredibly, Mum was undaunted. Instead of letting me watch regular television, she played hours and hours of videos showing me riding my motorbikes and snowboarding. She brought in my motorbike helmet and snowboard gear and stuck it all under my nose so I could smell the leather, the dirt, and the sweat. She surrounded my bed with extreme sports photos of me in action. She and Simon did everything possible to prevent me from mentally adjusting to life as a quadriplegic. Their objective was to help me visualize a return to everything that had previously given meaning to my life.

From Austin Hospital, I was transferred to the Royal Talbot Rehabilitation Centre where I encountered still more medical-establishment negativity. The way the physiotherapists saw it, their job was to help me psychologically adjust to life-in-a-wheelchair. I'll never forget being pushed in on a gurney at the Talbot through electronically-controlled doors. At that moment, I vowed: "Josh, you *will* walk out of this place under your own power!" Furthermore, I set my own timetable. With regular adjustments from Simon, non-stop motivation from Mum, and the heartfelt support of more friends than I ever realized I had, I left the Royal Talbot Rehabilitation Centre just days before my nineteenth birthday.

With discharge arrangements completed, I rolled to a point about four feet inside those electronically-controlled doors. I locked the brakes on my wheelchair, stood up unassisted, accepted the crutches my girlfriend handed me, and walked ten feet into the bright Melbourne sunshine while Mum captured every photo-album moment.

These events occurred ten years ago. Today, although I walk with a bit of a limp—and with the aid of a right-ankle brace and a walking stick—I manage to perform YouTube-posted stunts on my motorbike; ride a Harley; snowboard; and drive an automobile. To the bafflement of the medical establishment, my MRIs continue to show that ninety percent of my spinal cord is non-functional. Believe it or not, I'm still technically…"a quadriplegic!"

Through my passion for speed, I have experienced the desperate loneliness of severe spinal injury. And thanks to the body's Innate Intelligence in healing itself—largely facilitated by Chiropractic care, I have returned from that desolate island.

Joshua J. Wood
Chiropractic advocate and
Grateful quadriplegic patient of
Simon Floreani, DC
Vitality Chiropractic
Middle Park, Victoria
AUSTRALIA
As told to Don Dible

Dr. Simon Floreani served as
Technical Advisor on this story

12

Chiropractic Tributes

"Don't cry when the sun is gone
because the tears won't let you see the stars."

Violeta del Carmen Parra Sandoval
Chilean Folklorist
(1917-1967)

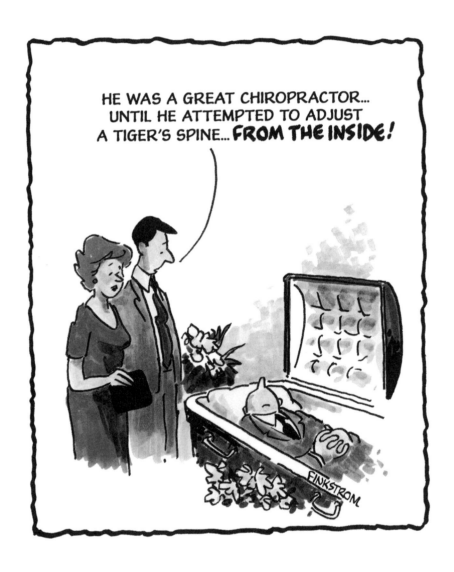

A Memory That Will Last a Lifetime

Elvie was a new patient who suffered from migraine headaches, dizziness, memory loss, and transient ischemic attacks (TIAs—temporary loss of blood to parts of the brain due to small clots) that were occurring with increasing frequency. Although her disposition was quite pleasant, you only had to look at her to appreciate that she was not in a "state of wellness."

While we pored over Elvie's medical history, it became increasingly apparent she was being treated for just about every "symptom" that could be clinically diagnosed. On the other hand, no attention had been given to treating "who she was." Elvie's list of medications included drugs for high blood pressure, high cholesterol, adult-onset diabetes, angina, migraines, pain, low blood sugar, and more. Most of the time, she was unable to do much because of fatigue and headaches. Sadly, she didn't want to get excited about anything because an elevated heart rate could trigger a stroke.

Further review of Elvie's lab work and a physical examination revealed that she was anemic, clinically hypoxic (not enough oxygen in her blood), a shallow breather with diminished rib motion, subluxated throughout her entire spine (almost all vertebra out of alignment), and exhibited forward head posture with increasing thoracic kyphosis (hunchback). In the previous three weeks, she had been in and out of the hospital six times. Following each release, she had been given a new set of prescriptions. Her medicine cabinet must have resembled a small pharmacy!

After our Chiropractic examination and consultation, I didn't have such a good feeling about what I thought I could do for Elvie. So, somewhere from within my soul, a question surfaced: "Elvie, what would you like me to do for you?"

In her sweetest and truest voice, she replied, "Dr. Mike, I would like to *sing* again."

"You would like to *sing* again?" I asked, not sure that I had heard correctly.

While reviewing Elvie's medical records and the results of her Chiropractic examination, I had momentarily lost sight of "who she was." Elvie was NOT merely a stack of x-rays, a list of medications, and a summary of "vital signs" scribbled on medical charts. What brought her the greatest joy in life was a passion for singing. Elvie simply wanted to be able to sing again.

After regaining my clinical composure, I focused on what it would take to enable Elvie to sing again. I decided that Chiropractic spinal adjustments, adjustments to her ribs, and a graduated exercise plan should do the trick. I saw Elvie six times over the course of a couple of weeks. During that period, I adjusted her lower neck, upper back, and ribs, procedures that significantly improved her breathing volumes. In turn, this reduced her migraines and TIA episodes by increasing oxygenation in her blood. Her oxygen saturations were increased from 89% to 94%. Additionally, soft tissue therapy was performed on her neck, upper back, and ribs. This afforded her more motion and freedom to allow her to perform more daily activities.

Weeks later, when Elvie was scheduled to return to our office, I noticed that she had cancelled her appointment. My first reaction was disappointment; but then it occurred to me that she might have had had a stroke and was in the hospital. My wife, also a chiropractor, called to determine Elvie's status and offered to reschedule her, if possible, since it was vital for her to stick to her treatment plan. Elvie did not say why she couldn't make her appointment other than that she would try to get in the following week.

It was another three weeks before Elvie finally returned to our office. When I heard her voice coming from the reception area, I realized that I was truly "happy" to know she was there. I went out and greeted her, saying that I'd be with her shortly.

With a little girl look on her face, Elvie announced that she had something for me.

"What is it?" I asked.

She shyly held out a freshly-minted CD filled with her singing. Two lines on the jewel case label proclaimed, "Thank you God" and "Thank You Dr. Hall."

I could not contain my emotions as I was reminded of just how important it is to know "what people want" in today's world. For Elvie, she just wanted to sing. I told her, "Sing forever! Don't stop!"

That day, Elvie gave me not only a CD, she gave me a "Memory That Will Last a Lifetime." She reawakened in me awareness of exactly why I had chosen Chiropractic as my life's work—to help sick people get well.

Dr. James W. Parker first instilled that principle in me in 1987 when I began my studies at the Parker College of Chiropractic. Twenty years later, Elvie allowed me "to live" that principle. With faith in my God, the love and support of my family, and the memory of Elvie, I continue my mission in "helping sick people get well."

Michael W. Hall, DC, FIACN
Hall Chiropractic and Neurology Center
Cedar Hill, Texas

Professor /Chiropractic Neurologist
Parker College of Chiropractic
Dallas, Texas

Paying Tribute to a Hero

"When I call your name,
would you be the same,
if I see you in heaven?"

Eric Clapton
English rock music artist

In America, we've come to define heroes as people who have braved difficult circumstances—sacrificed themselves—to benefit others and serve a purpose that was pure and selfless.

Recently, one of my heroes passed away. Her name was Cheryl Jean. To me, Cheryl Jean and her parents personify the term "hero."

For the last six years of her life, Cheryl Jean fought leukemia. She never gave up—even in her last breath. This ten-year-old little angel-on-earth cherished every second of every day. She managed to give smiles to everyone she met, even when her body and insides were screaming in pain. Cheryl Jean displaced her own personal turmoil by redirecting her attention to helping others feel better. She didn't know this consciously, but it was obvious.

We all should learn from the lessons Cheryl Jean taught us: "Cherish every moment," and "Consider others first."

Cheryl Jean got Chiropractic adjustments throughout her entire term of illness. Chiropractic ignited the life energy in her, and she lit up the room after every treatment. She was exceptionally receptive to the healing that occurred each time her nervous system was re-balanced. She would allow the restored life force to enter every cell of her body.

We finished every treatment with a long bear hug. I learned to make simple balloon animals for Cheryl Jean since she loved them and they brought smiles to her face. This was part of our treatment ritual. We chiropractors know that it's not always just the hands-on touching that heals our patients, but the touching of soul-to-soul. It's the little, extraordinary things we do that turn a child's life on and make massive positive changes in their healing and general outlook.

Cheryl Jean wanted to be home in her own bed with her own teddy bears on her last night on earth. She also asked that I be present as she passed on. Never was I so privileged and honored as a chiropractor, let alone a human being, than to share these transformational moments. Cheryl Jean was in pain and gasping for air as her mom, dad, and I held her hands and comforted her. Our eyes locked, and I knew she had come to peace. What an amazing, courageous child!

For Cheryl Jean's parents, it was six years of unconditional love. We sometimes forget about the caretakers of these children who are going through the battle. I wish to acknowledge Linda and John for demonstrating the true meaning of unconditional love. They sacrificed everything to make their child's every moment more comfortable. In doing so, they created a bond that many parents can only dream about.

Linda and John exemplify the relationship we all could have with our kids if we put our hearts and souls into it. They may have lost their daughter after only ten years, but the bond they had with her will last an eternity. I thank them for reminding me how short life is and how every moment with your children should be quality time, not just occasionally.

Heroes exist to set the bar just a little higher for the rest of us. Heroes show us personality traits to emulate. I will miss Cheryl Jean's bear hugs, but I will remember her every time I see another human being and smile. Part of that smile will belong to Cheryl Jean.

My relationship with Cheryl Jean personifies how Chiropractic is demonstrated in the greater scheme of life. Touching lives to make their quality better and more harmonious, even if for a short moment, changes our world.

Steven J. Pollack, DC
Pollack Health and Wellness
Beachwood, New Jersey

Dr. Pollack is the author of
Ask the Chiropractor I and *II*

Bon Appétit

While in Chiropractic College, I once heard a professor say, "Treat regular folk as if they are famous people and famous people like they're regular folk." The first half of that advice served me well for years, but then I met Graham Kerr.

While the new patient was filling out a few forms in my reception room, I recognized a pleasant English accent, but the name Graham Kerr made no impact on me at all. That was until my wife asked in hushed tones, *"Do you know who* that *is?"* Before I could recall the name I'd been given, she swooned, exclaiming, *"That's 'The Galloping Gourmet'!"*

As a youngster, I remember sitting before the television set, totally entertained by this culinary giant. Perhaps it was my mother who tuned in, but I was captivated as this witty young man chopped, diced, and sautéed his way into our living room. Never could I have imagined that someday he would literally walk into *my* adjusting room!

It's hard to imagine Kerr as anything but a gourmet chef buzzing about an immaculate studio kitchen, creating dishes to please both the eye and the palate. Yet, when asked what first led him to a chiropractor, he related a surprising story of an injury sustained while he was a commissioned officer in the Royal New Zealand Air Force.

The year was 1960. Strong winds make the Wellington Straights a favorite site for sailing in New Zealand. However, the Straights are also known for sudden southerly storms with terrifying gale winds.

A small sailboat, transporting a couple and their young child, could not make it to safety as the winds picked up one day. Large waves began to smash the boat against the rocks along the shore.

Squadron Leader Kerr participated in the rescue, helping the family ashore without incident. However, in the process, he slipped on a rock—slick with lichens and sea spray—and fell.

The injuries resulting from the fall caused him excruciating back pain. Every doctor on the military base took his turn at trying to correct the young officer's problem. Their treatment consisted of recommending bed rest, prescribing painkillers, and even having him lie down on boards. No course of care eased Kerr's discomfort. Finally, a doctor who specialized in treating injuries sustained by downed pilots during World War II visited Kerr's bedside. The specialist utilized adjustments of the vertebrae to restore proper function to the spine. Within a short period, Kerr's symptoms began to subside. Eventually, his recovery was complete, and Graham Kerr has been a fan of Chiropractic ever since.

In the early period of New Zealand's television industry, the Air Force broadcast a daily physical fitness program. One day, the drill sergeant who led the activity didn't show up on time. Since the program was a live broadcast, a senior officer ordered Kerr to appear on television in the drill sergeant's place.

As the *Chief Catering Advisor* to the Air Force, Kerr didn't feel qualified to lead TV viewers in exercise. So that day, no vigorous workout was broadcast. Instead, Kerr treated the audience to his spontaneity and humor while preparing a delicious omelet. His TV debut was in uniform, with no apron—still his trademark cooking attire.

It was after a successful national cooking show in Australia that Kerr moved to Canada to film "The Galloping Gourmet," a show that caught the world's attention and quickly became the most successful cooking program on television. Behind every great man is a great woman and Kerr's wife, Treena, received two Emmy nominations as producer of his daytime television show.

Then tragedy struck. In 1971, a vegetable truck crashed into Kerr's on-location production vehicle near San Francisco,

California. Graham was paralyzed on his left side, and Treena suffered complications that required major surgery.

The Kerrs devoted the next two years to rehabilitation and reordering their lives. After returning to their native country, England, they stayed at the Forest Mere Health Hydro, a world-famous health spa that was featured in the James Bond film, "Thunderball." From a Chiropractic perspective, the most interesting scene in the movie is when the undercover spy, Bond (Sean Connery), is given a brief massage by a beautiful female therapist who proceeds to manipulate every bone in his spine.

Fortunately, Graham Kerr's care was a bit milder than that given to the secret agent. In a short time, Graham's paralysis abated; but he still had a problem with dizziness. Literally, he would fall down after eating meals.

A Scottish doctor prescribed a sea voyage for him. The expectation was that the motion of the boat would challenge Kerr's sense of balance; and the rigor of life aboard a sailboat was sure to help him regain his strength.

For two years, the Kerrs sailed with their three children 24,000 miles across the Atlantic and throughout the Caribbean. Fully recovered and fit once again after this journey, the family returned to the United States.

Soon after a conversion to Christianity led the Kerrs to focus their talents toward helping the less fortunate, it was Treena's heart attack that motivated Graham to put his new lifestyle and cooking technique on television. He saw the need to reduce the dangerous properties of traditional, high-fat cooking without reducing its enjoyment, creativity, or taste.

Reflected in each of Kerr's endeavors is one thing that always stands out: He loves people and has an interest and compassion for others. He is naturally at ease with people, and for years I enjoyed watching him chat and laugh candidly with other patients in my reception room. Food may be his business, but it is clear that *people* are his true delight. Obviously, in Kerr's mind, *everybody* is a famous person.

I'm not certain whether it's his past injuries, his healthy lifestyle, or his busy schedule that has made Graham Kerr appreciate the value of Chiropractic most. No matter the reason, the man who shows the world how to create "Great Food for Great Years" knows that regular Chiropractic adjustments are essential.

Ray Pope, DC
Action Potential Chiropractic
Camano Island, Washington

Lesley's Story

Dedication

This story is dedicated to Lesley Camisa, Chiropractic Assistant, who was taken from us very suddenly due to complications arising from breast cancer.

Christie MacDonald, DC

Chiropractic is unique in the healing arts, not only in its approach to health and wellness, but in allowing patients to feel acknowledged and valued in a warm, welcoming, and educating environment.

Lesley Camisa joined our team in September 2001. We loved her energy from the moment we met her. Warm and caring, she had a very charming Welsh accent. Although she knew nothing about Chiropractic when she first joined our clinic, she told us she wanted to try something new and possibly make a difference in the world. Well, that is exactly what Lesley did.

For seven years, Lesley's smiling face was the very first thing that greeted patients as they entered the office of Whitemud Crossing Chiropractors. She made a point of talking to, and getting to know, each and every patient. She listened as they explained what had brought them to the office. Visitors told her stories about their children and grandchildren and brought pictures from their most recent holidays, weddings, or births. She became an integral part of the healing process in our office. Lesley made everyone feel loved and listened to and was well known for being able to calm down the most upset of babies. When the other Chiropractic Assistants were handed a crying baby that no one could settle, the infant was immediately passed on to "Grandma" Lesley. Within minutes, you could hear cooing coming from the front office.

Lesley was as reliable as clockwork and never missed a beat as she helped with whatever the doctors, patients, or other Chiropractic Assistants needed. Always upbeat, she transformed even the most challenging people and situations into positive experiences. Lesley was excited to learn the philosophy and principles of Chiropractic. She was fascinated to learn about the body's innate ability to heal itself, and the power of the nervous system and how it controls and regulates every cell, tissue and organ in the body. She was amazed by the miracles she saw in the office on a daily basis. Lesley was especially intrigued when she witnessed the recovery of a man who presented at the clinic with debilitating arm pain and severe muscle atrophy. Unable to work for months due to pain, he had been told by his medical doctors that his only option for relief was neck surgery. As a last resort, a friend referred him to our office. After about a month of Chiropractic care, he began to use his arm again; the function of his nervous system had been restored.

Lesley watched the progress of babies that were unable to sleep, or who were colicky, as their bodies responded to Chiropractic with the calming result that they were able to enjoy hours of healing rest. Seniors, originally scheduled for knee replacements, cancelled their surgeries as their knee pain was relieved. A middle-aged man who loved golf used Chiropractic as his secret weapon to enhance his game, thus enjoying a competitive advantage over his golfing buddies. The nervous system—and subsequently, the immune system—of a child suffering from chronic bladder infections for most of her young life were restored through Chiropractic. Lesley observed all of these transformations and was thrilled and amazed by what she saw.

Lesley helped change the lives of hundreds of people—not only from her duties as a Chiropractic Assistant, but also by referring people in need to Chiropractic care. When she heard about a friend, mother, or child that was experiencing a health complaint, she would explain to them that Chiropractic may be able to help. One woman, suffering with severe constipation issues for years, had consulted many medical doctors and had tried all the conventional medical protocols. When this woman checked in at our center, she told Lesley that her doctors were recommending the surgical removal of part of her bowel to remedy the constipation and severe abdominal pain. To make matters worse, the doctors would not guarantee that the pain would be gone after surgery. The patient is now under Chiropractic care and is benefiting from this natural approach to health.

Lesley applied the principles she learned in the office to her own life. She enjoyed walking with her husband, Ray, and included daily physical activity as an integral aspect of the Chiropractic lifestyle. Lesley and Ray both received adjustments on a regular basis, and they strove to maintain a healthy balance in their lives. The couple laughed a lot, and they traveled whenever they could. Both of them valued and enjoyed time with their three grown children—visiting, playing games, and laughing.

Two weeks before she was taken from us, Lesley just happened to be in the right place at the right time to help a group of seniors. She and her husband were awakened at three in the morning by the shriek of a fire alarm. As they departed their building, they were horrified to see a massive blaze on the roof of the seniors' complex next door. The elderly were pouring out into the cold with only robes and slippers to protect them from the harsh winter elements. Thinking quickly, Leslie approached a fireman and said that although she didn't want to interfere, she did have a key to the Chiropractic office just across the street and could provide shelter. After he was assured that there was plenty of room, he sent over a large group of shivering, frightened, newly-homeless seniors with her until other arrangements could be made. Lesley sent Ray back home to get a large tray of cookies they had bought earlier in the day. Leslie witnessed the need, rose to the occasion, and distributed warmth, compassion, and cookies to her guests. A news reporter from a local television station interviewed Lesley in the clinic that early morning. In his broadcast, he mentioned how impressive it was that the neighborhood pulled together to display many acts of kindness. In her customary, straightforward manner, Lesley responded, "You can't just leave people out in the cold." We were so proud of Lesley for her proactive part in responding to this dire situation.

Our profession is different; often that is realized the moment a patient walks in the door of any Chiropractic office. Patients should feel they are cared for, that they matter, and that the clinic has a genuine interest in getting them healthy. Lesley embodied all this and more. Her positive effect on patients was tremendous and that was evident when Lesley passed away so suddenly. Our patients seemed to feel as though they had lost someone very significant in their lives. Patients were devastated and emotional, and generously offered support to Lesley's family and all our office personnel.

Lesley demonstrated just how important the Chiropractic Assistant (CA) is, not only to answer the phone and book appointments, but also as the first and last person a patient will see in the office. CAs are an important piece of the puzzle, contributing to the health and wellness of the patients. They serve as educators on the benefits of ongoing wellness care. They serve as ambassadors for the Chiropractic lifestyle. And they see first-hand the miracles of Chiropractic.

Lesley Camisa was an angel. We were blessed to have her in our lives; and the lessons we learned from her were invaluable. She will be dearly missed.

Christie MacDonald, DC
Whitemud Crossing Chiropractors
Edmonton, Alberta
CANADA

My Father: The Chiropractor Who Helped Millions

"Once you start giving, there is no lack of anything."

Monte H. Greenawalt, DC, DABCO
Founder of Foot Levelers, Inc.
(1923-2007)

The life story of my father, Dr. Monte H. Greenawalt, is one of faith, love and service. He had an abiding faith that God had a plan for him, and that faith instilled a confidence in his ability to serve mankind. My father's story of success is remarkable, not because of what he achieved, but because of *how he chose to turn adversity into opportunity* time and time again. The speed bumps he hit in life only fueled him to work harder and focus on helping other people.

At so many stages of my father's life, adversity led to opportunity. A child of the Great Depression, he raised and sold vegetables in his neighborhood in order to help his family. He organized a local lawn and home-care service when he was in high school, and by the time he was a senior he had added a car business to his list of enterprises. He gave half of what he earned to his family and ten percent to his church.

After the Japanese attack on Pearl Harbor, my father signed up to go into the military. Of course, to enlist, you had to go through a series of examinations and physicals to make sure you were fit to go to war overseas. In the process of going through that examination, my dad received some inoculations; and unfortunately, the bad vaccine he received actually killed about 150 people. Although it didn't *kill* my father, it caused paralysis—forcing him to wear an iron lung (a medical device used to do the breathing for you). Dad lay in that iron lung for six months! He told people he would lie there for half an hour just trying to move his little finger. The effort would cause him to break into a cold sweat; and no matter how hard he tried, he just couldn't move.

On hearing the news that he'd spend the rest of his life as a paraplegic, my dad asked God to let him die...but God had other plans. Not long afterward, Dad accepted the fact that he *wasn't* going to die, so he decided to offer God a proposition: "Let me walk again and I'll devote the rest of my life to helping people."

One day, his mother (my grandmother) said the family was going to try something different, so he was taken to a chiropractor. *"They* carried *him in and he* walked *out!"* is how my grandmother described what happened. It was literally a miracle!

As a young man, my father had planned to be a neurosurgeon, but he believed there was a message in this miracle. He said, "Chiropractic is a wonderful profession; and I want to be a part of it." That's how the seed was planted for the birth of his practice (and later, for the birth of his company, Foot Levelers).

When Dr. Greenawalt began his Chiropractic practice in 1948, the only office space he could lay his hands on was in the basement of a bank in Dubuque, Iowa. It must not have seemed like the perfect place to start at the time. Not only was he beginning below the ground floor, but the basement needed remodeling.

This was not a promising start for a young chiropractor. Dr. Greenawalt needed equipment and office furniture before he could treat patients, and he didn't have the money to pay for them. It could have been an occasion for hopelessness, but Dr.

Greenawalt had faith. He decided to take direct action instead and paid a visit to the bank upstairs.

When the talking was over, the bankers had agreed not only to make the necessary improvements in the office space, but also agreed to lend him the money needed to buy equipment. Now, Dr. Greenawalt's practice of Chiropractic had begun.

Next door to his office was a podiatrist, and the two doctors regularly referred patients to each other. Dad would refer patients with foot problems to the podiatrist, and the podiatrist would give them hard-arch supports to wear in their shoes. My dad noticed that many times when those same patients came back for a Chiropractic adjustment, their condition was worse and their adjustment wouldn't hold very long. Adjustments were supposed to *improve* with those supports! So my father reasoned that if foot supports can have a negative effect, then properly-designed foot supports should produce a positive effect.

Dad started a series of experiments—mostly through trial and error—to determine what could be done to make the ultimate, custom-made orthotic (shoe insert) for the patient. As a result of his investigations, he came upon what he called "the correct way to support the foot." He discovered that it was necessary to support all three arches to have optimal results. Afterward, his patient's adjustments held longer. His patients felt better. And right there, the first Spinal Pelvic Stabilizer was born.

In Dad's practice, which had become quite successful, he and his growing staff were now seeing about 200-250 patients a day. He went from working in the basement of a bank to buying an old school building in which to operate his clinic. Next to the school was a carriage house (like a small garage) and that's where he created Stabilizers for his patients. That carriage house is where Foot Levelers was born.

In 1968—twenty years after starting his practice—Dr. Greenawalt was seriously injured in an automobile accident. Unable to work for two years, he could do nothing but lie on his bed. Events such as this have been turning points in many lives, though not often for the better. By this time, Dr. Greenawalt had gone too far in his habits of success to spend his time unproductively. Instead, he developed ideas and communicated those ideas to others by phone. Even while laid-up in bed, he kept trying to be of service.

When he was a little better, Dr. Greenawalt returned to the business of giving lectures and seminars around the country. In his efforts to help doctors give better service to their patients, he spoke from his own experience on orthopedics and on how to manage a Chiropractic practice. He passed along the benefit of his experience to thousands of doctors and their assistants.

Dad used to tell others, "Every night, I say to myself, 'My creative mind will come forth with new and productive ideas.'" It worked. The ideas kept coming for him—out of his own experience and fuelled by his desire to help others.

For example, one inspiration came to him on a plane as he was returning home from a seminar. He was experiencing considerable pain from his auto accident injuries and was unable to get comfortable. From this discomfort came a therapeutic traction device—a uniquely-designed bed pillow.

That was my father: a man who always had faith in himself and his abilities to help others, even in the face of seemingly insurmountable obstacles. A firm advocate of "planning your work and working your plan," Dad put great stock in the effectiveness of visualizing your goals and writing them down. He thought about his goals constantly!

Thanks to my dad's vision, Foot Levelers has become a worldwide company that has provided custom-made Spinal Pelvic Stabilizers—and many other innovative healthcare products—to millions of patients. My dad spent a lifetime helping people, and that help continues today through the Monte H. Greenawalt Foundation which has donated millions of dollars to help patients through Chiropractic care.

When Dr. Monte passed away at the age of 84, I was touched by the thousands of heartfelt stories people shared with me of how my dad affected their lives in a positive way. *And that, to me, is his legacy.*

Kent S. Greenawalt
President and CEO
Foot Levelers, Inc.
Roanoke, Virginia

13

The Golden Years

"Beautiful young people are accidents of nature,
but beautiful old people are works of art."

Anna Eleanor Roosevelt
First Lady of the United States (1933-1945)
Writer, Humanitarian, Chair,
United Nations committee that drafted and approved the
Universal Declaration of Human Rights
Niece of President Theodore Roosevelt
(1884-1962)

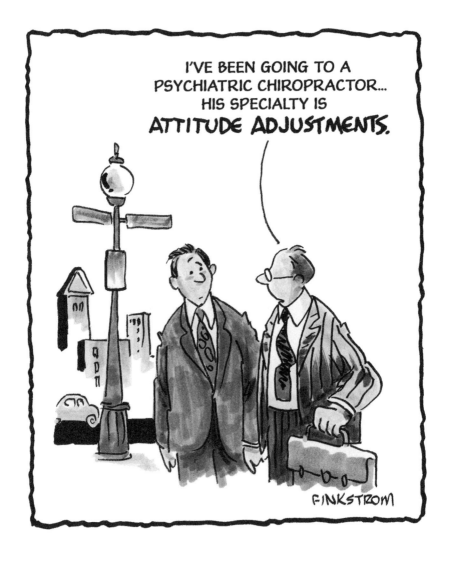

Reprinted by arrangement with Finkstrom Licensing International

The Healing of Three Generations

Dorothy, a fellow-Montanan, was 66 when she first came to see me. You could say that she was *dragged* in—kicking and screaming—by her sister who was very concerned about her sibling's health. Weighing only 79 pounds and barely able to walk on her own, Dorothy was struggling to survive after a devastating car accident seven years earlier. Lucky to still be alive, Dorothy barely had the stamina to make it through a typical day dominated, as they *all* were, by excruciating pain and depression.

Ever skeptical, Dorothy swore to her sister that she would not return to my office after her first visit provided no immediate relief. Her sister refused to let her give up and stated in no uncertain terms that she *would* be returning for further care. Dorothy relented and proceeded with her treatments. After only the third visit, the world suddenly saw a *new* Dorothy! She couldn't believe it! She could *walk*, she could *breathe*, and she felt like she was *living* again instead of *merely surviving*. In three short months, she weighed a healthy 110 pounds and started telling everyone about the wonders of Chiropractic. Today, Dorothy says she has more stamina than one retired grandma needs, so she's sharing her newfound energy through a new job at the local Boys and Girls Club.

Dorothy was so happy with her new quality of life that she asked if I could possibly do something to help her son who lived in Wyoming. I said I'd be honored to see him the next time he came to visit. When Donald first dropped in at my office, he'd already had a cancerous right kidney removed and—two years later—was suffering from what his medical doctors deemed "terminal" and "inoperable" lung cancer. I told Donald that we would certainly do what we could. He began to travel back and forth on a regular basis for care and—almost immediately—noticed improvements in his quality of life. The chronic migraine headaches that he used to suffer vanished. He started sleeping better. He got off the slippery slope of steady weight loss and anemia and started putting healthy muscle back on his wasted frame! His latest CAT scan revealed no new cancer growth and—though he's only been in Chiropractic for a few months—Donald is confident he's winning the battle with "terminal" lung cancer. Of course, he attributes this amazing turnaround to Chiropractic.

Dorothy, seeing the clear-cut improvements in her own health and that of her son, decided to add yet a third generation to my patient list: little Randy, her grandson. The next time Donald and his young family made the trek from Wyoming to Montana, he brought his five-year-old into my office. Although Randy's earliest years seemed "almost normal" to his parents, the boy's motor skills were slow to develop. They had taken Randy to see numerous medical doctors and specialists, but got no satisfaction. Finally, when he was just two, a specialist diagnosed him as "autistic." By the time I saw Randy—three years after his "autistic" diagnosis, he had become extremely withdrawn and appeared to have no ability whatsoever at social interaction. His parents told me he didn't ever speak or smile. He clung to his father or tried to hide in the corner through most of our visit. I was pretty sure that the boy was still suffering from subluxations caused by birth trauma. I adjusted Randy every day for about a week until his family had to return to Wyoming.

The next time the family made a visit to see grandma, they brought Randy into our office. My staff and I were delighted to "meet" a totally new human being! Randy was smiling and talking. He greeted us with a boisterous *"Hello!"* His parents told us he was able to count to 10 and could recite his ABCs. My Chiropractic

Assistants immediately fell in love with Randy and he returned their affection with hugs and kisses. We still see Randy on a regular basis, and he is continually improving. Dorothy says he's even learning how to make his "Papa" coffee and loves to give everyone he meets BIG hugs. What could be better than that?

It's wonderful to see Chiropractic affect a life in such a profound way, but to see it touch and change *three generations* suffering more heartache than any one family should have to bear, well, that's truly a testament to the miraculous healing power of Chiropractic!

Erik H. Norslien, DC
Lewistown, Montana

Chiropractic First, Not Last!

*"Tears of joy are like
the summer rain drops
pierced by sunbeams."*

Hosea Ballou
American Universalist clergyman
and theological writer
(1771-1852)

I've practiced in the Ozark foothills for the past 31 years where it has been my privilege to serve the good folks of Greers Ferry, Arkansas. The first time I met Mrs. McClintock, I observed a medium-framed, slightly-overweight lady who grimaced in pain with each tentative step she took.

During our consultation, she recited her case history in a monotone pretty much as she had with numerous medical doctors during the previous seven years. She'd been hit from behind in a seemingly-minor car accident. Although there wasn't much damage to either vehicle, her head did whip backwards against the headrest, and she experienced immediate neck pain. She went to the local emergency room where x-rays were taken. Since no bones were broken, she was sent home with pain pills and told she'd be fine. Over the next few days, in spite of her following the orders of the hospital medical doctor, her pain steadily worsened.

Mrs. McClintock then visited her family medical doctor in the hope of securing relief. She was told she had a simple strain—a strain of the neck, and that she should continue taking her pain pills and use a heating pad. "You'll be fine in a few days," she was told. But as time passed, the pain continued to worsen; she began to lose the use of her left arm as it was overtaken by a steadily-increasing numbness.

Later, she was referred to an orthopedist. He ordered more x-rays and a very painful myelogram where a contrast agent was injected through a needle into the space around her spinal cord to display the spinal cord, spinal canal, and nerve roots. After studying the new x-rays, her orthopedist prescribed steroids and told Mrs. McClintock she'd be fine in no time.

While all this happened over a three-year period, Mrs. McClintock was transformed from a vibrant, rather slim, regularly-exercising, middle-aged woman into a creature doomed to sleepless nights and excruciating neck and low-back pain. She gained forty pounds. During this interval, she was shuffled from neurologists to pain doctors and back to neurologists, none of whom provided relief.

Near the end of our initial Chiropractic consultation, Mrs. McClintock described her final visit with a neurologist. He told her that he could possibly do surgery and cut several of the nerves in her neck to relieve *some* of the pain. When asked if he thought this would permanently correct her problem and give her back the use of her arm, the neurologist replied, "To be honest, I don't know! *Your pain might even get worse!*"

With her long history of medical doctor visits, I couldn't resist asking why she finally decided to try Chiropractic. She said her neighbor was a patient of mine, had attended our spinal health care class, and had learned about the adverse effects of subluxations of the spine. Mrs. McClintock's neighbor told her, "Your problems *could* be coming from a spinal subluxation, and I'm sure my chiropractor can help!"

Upon examination, I found a very swollen and painful area in her neck that had likely been there for a long time. During the Report of Findings, I explained to Mrs. McClintock and her husband that her x-rays revealed vertebral subluxations in her neck and low back. When I asked if she was aware of this, she replied, "No one has ever found that before." I further explained that these subluxations, over time, had been the cause of the pain and muscle degeneration she had experienced. I then reviewed a treatment program appropriate for her problem.

In closing my Report of Findings, I asked if she had any questions. With a smile and look of hope she replied, "You've found my problem and it's a *subluxation!* I knew *someone* could identify my problem and determine that I wasn't crazy!"

Mr. McClintock asked me how long it would take for his wife to finally get well. I responded that each person heals at a different rate, and that I'd perform periodic examinations to monitor her progress. I told him I'd guarantee one thing—if we didn't see the results I anticipated, I'd tell them straight away. I wouldn't have her coming in for adjustments if we weren't making progress.

We began her initial phase of care with a spinal adjustment. She stated she immediately had more movement in her neck. She returned two days later and reported with amazement, "I slept better during the past two nights than I have in the past two years!" With each visit, she had good news to report: decreased pain, increased movement. Her arm felt less tingly and had increased strength. "I was able to lift my grandchild for the first time in two years, and I could even open her baby food jar without help!" We celebrated each and every improvement.

During the corrective phase of care, most of her pain decreased substantially. We began to make permanent changes to her spine and nervous system. One day, I entered the adjusting room to find Mrs. McClintock in tears. My mind reeled with apprehensive curiosity. Had she had another accident? A relapse? She turned her head and looked at me—a movement she could not perform prior to the start of treatment. She held a photo of herself taken shortly after her accident. It showed a face contorted in agony reflecting the pain she subsequently endured for seven years. "Dr. Carnathan, look at this picture. I could have been this way *the rest of my life* if someone hadn't told me about Chiropractic. *Now look at me!*" She then turned her head from side to side, raised both arms above her head, and reached toward me for a hug!

The body is self-healing and self-correcting. When the spinal subluxation is removed, the body is allowed to heal. Want proof? Just ask Mrs. McClintock!

Alan B. Carnathan, DC
Carnathan Chiropractic Clinic
Greers Ferry, Arkansas

Mrs. Nasty becomes Mrs. Nice

My wife, Lois, and I are both chiropractors. When we first started our practice, we had a lot more time than patients. So we decided to volunteer once a week to deliver "Meals on Wheels" to the elderly. Our regular destination was a convalescent home located in a downtown high-rise. One of our clients, who lived on the eleventh floor, was an elderly woman in her 90s by the name of Mrs. Nice. This person could not have been more inappropriately named. She was so crabby that we secretly called her Mrs. Nasty! We'd walk into her apartment and always find her sitting bolt upright in a corner chair—with a sinister look in her eyes and a scowl on her lips. She actually grunted at us as a means of replying to almost any question we asked from, "How are you today?" to "Did you do anything nice for the weekend?"

Well, as we got to know Mrs. Nice a little better, and developed the ability to interpret her grunts, we realized that she had good reason to be crotchety. She had rarely been out of her apartment in years because of chronic back, neck, and foot pain. She sat in the same corner, not really wanting visitors, and got around with the aid of her walker only when necessary.

After we had delivered meals to her for a couple of months, Lois asked if she would like to be adjusted. When we explained a few simple Chiropractic principles—like having an innate intelligence within, and her body's ability to heal once her nervous system was free of interference, and finally, describing how gentle our adjustments would be—she agreed, but not without some apprehension.

We started bringing our portable adjusting table with us; and, for the following several weeks, gave her an adjustment along with her meal. At first, after each adjustment, she'd work herself up off the table, grunt, and then laboriously make her way back to the corner chair with the help of her walker. It wasn't long, however, before she sensed something positive was happening because she would—voluntarily and without assistance—get back on the table each time we set it up on the following visit.

About two months after her first adjustment, we entered Mrs. Nice's apartment and found a vaguely familiar woman sitting in her chair. She looked *something* like the previous occupant except that this woman had a smile on her face and was wearing lipstick and blush. Also, this woman had on a dress instead of a tattered housecoat. She convinced us that it was really her and began to describe trips up and down the hall that she had been taking for exercise. She then excitedly detailed her foray downstairs the day before to visit old friends in the recreation room. It had been her first visit there in a couple of years.

Through Chiropractic, this lonely lady had regained *some* of her health and *a lot* of her smile. We couldn't call Mrs. Nice Mrs. Nasty anymore!

George B. Donnelly, DC
Birmingham, Alabama

Adam's Apple: Front-and-Center!

This is not your typical Chiropractic success story where the patient comes in after years of suffering, learns the Big Idea about Chiropractic, gets adjusted, has a dramatic change in their health, and goes on to live the rest of their life in happiness and health.... Or is it?

John was referred to me by his massage therapist and his family physician, both of whom are patients of mine. They thought that Chiropractic might be of some assistance to the man. My new patient was seventy and looked every day as old as his three-score-and-ten years. A retired professor at a nearby university, he had obviously never made any effort to care for his health. John's reason for consulting my office was that he was experiencing a lot of leg and arm discomfort—constant and rated in the range of eight-to-nine on a pain scale of ten! As might be expected, his medical doctors had provided John with numerous pain medications, and he had relied on these for relief over a period of many years. Although he could stand; he wasn't able to walk and got around by riding a motorized scooter.

On John's first visit, I performed a standard Chiropractic analysis that included a physical examination as well as a scan of the spine to show me how his nerves and muscles were functioning. We also x-rayed his neck and lumbar spine (lower back).

On reviewing the information I had gathered on the initial exam, it was clear that John was not only having significant, constant pain in his legs and arms; but that he was, overall, not a very healthy gentleman. John's skin was pale; his breathing was labored; and he just didn't look well. Our x-rays revealed severe degenerative changes, both in his neck and lower back— major factors contributing to the pain he was experiencing in his arms and legs. In addition, his bone density was very low, indicating that he was also afflicted with osteoporosis.

The next day when John came to my office for his Report of Findings, I showed him his x-rays and scans. I told him that his pain was unquestionably due to problems in his spine. I also explained that his steadily-diminishing health had been going on for a very long time due to severe degenerative changes. The onset of osteoporosis further complicated matters. I also explained that if we got pressure off the nervous system, his brain would better be able to communicate with the tissue cells and that he *might* have a reduction in pain.

Given the advanced state of John's ill-health, I was quick to add that I wasn't sure *precisely* how much I'd be able to help him. I told him that the Innate Intelligence of his body—that had created him some seventy years earlier—was what was going to get him well as long as we could restore the pathways for messages flowing down his spinal cord. John, obviously a very smart man, seemed quite intrigued by his scans, my discussion of the benefits of Chiropractic care, and the role of Innate Intelligence in the healing process. Or, perhaps, he was simply looking desperately for a ray of hope. Major pain has been known to trigger that, you know.

I suggested that we do a trial of Chiropractic care and, after an eight-week period, we'd discuss his progress and determine if we should continue. I also told John that, due to his severe arthritis and osteoporosis, I wouldn't be administering my typical treatments by hand alone. Instead, I'd provide a combination of hand adjustments augmented by the use of a special instrument that would give a small push to his vertebrae that were subluxated. He seemed eager to begin and immediately booked sixteen appointments over the next eight weeks.

To be honest, I wasn't that confident in John's ability to get better, but he was committed for eight weeks, so I assured him I'd do everything in my power to help him. After several visits, he started to feel a little better in his arms and legs. He reported that he felt a bit stronger. On his re-evaluation at the eight-week mark, we measured modest improvement in his scans. Furthermore, he said he was feeling decidedly stronger and had less pain. John also indicated that he no longer was incontinent each night, an embarrassing problem with which he had suffered for a number of years in spite of taking a prescribed medication. He confessed that he'd initially been too ashamed to tell me he wore diapers to bed. I reiterated what I'd told John at his Report of Findings: the relief he was experiencing made sense considering the areas of subluxation that had been adjusted in his spine. Needless to say, he began to look better and got some color in his cheeks. His breathing was less labored as well. We decided to continue on a two-treatments-per-week basis since he was experiencing modest-but-noticeable improvements after each visit.

A couple of weeks later at one of his scheduled appointments, John seemed to be looking more pleased than usual. Although he was still using his scooter to get around, at home he'd also make use of his walker to move from room-to-room. In fact, as he felt stronger, he'd actually take a couple of steps to get from his scooter to the table. John smiled at me and said, "Look at this!" pointing to the front of his neck. I looked curiously.... "Yes, its *straight!*" he proclaimed. "My Adam's apple is *in the middle of my neck!*" John went on to explain that when he was a little boy playing on a high pile of snow in the schoolyard, another child had pushed him and caused him to fall. Ever since that day, his Adam's apple had been off to the side. I hadn't even noticed that before, nor did my treatments ever go anywhere near his throat! (My efforts had been confined exclusively to adjusting subluxations in his spine.) John's Innate Intelligence was producing all the healing and positive changes that were going on.

Over the next few weeks, John continued to watch his body and see improvements in his digestion, breathing, pain levels, etc. Then, one day, he caught a cold and said he was feeling worn down. The symptoms continued for a couple of weeks, so he went to his family medical doctor who confirmed it was just a cold and that he should be feeling better soon...but he didn't. One day, he collapsed and was rushed from home to hospital by ambulance. Shortly thereafter, John died due to a strange blood infection.

Of course, I was shocked and saddened when I heard the news. I was also a little nervous as my assistant told me John's wife was on the phone and wanted to speak with me. I felt a bit queasy and had a lump in my throat as I picked up the receiver. I gave her my condolences, and she thanked me. But she also thanked me for what I had done for her husband. She said that John had been sick and in great pain for many years, and that he had really come to believe in Chiropractic. Even though he had been under my care for just a few months, it had made a big difference in the quality of his life, and she thought I should know that.

As I sat in my office after hanging up, I wondered what difference Chiropractic could have made in John's life if he'd known about it sooner—and if he still would be alive today. What if he had gotten adjusted shortly after being pushed off that high pile of snow as a young boy? What differences would that have made in his health and his life?

These are questions that nobody can answer. John taught me never to underestimate the power of the body to heal. More importantly, he reaffirmed my belief that the sooner we look after ourselves, the longer we'll be able to enjoy a quality life.

Michael G. Staffen, DC
Sudbury Chiropractic & Wellness Centre
Sudbury, Ontario
CANADA

Emma's High-Flying Adjustment

"Is there a doctor on board? If so, please press your call button."

The announcement stirred me from sleep in my reclined airplane seat. I listened and, again, the request was repeated with more information: "We have an elderly woman in distress who's having trouble breathing." I hesitated a moment, then reached up and pressed the call button.

A flight attendant came back to my seat and asked how I could help. I told her I was a chiropractor with some emergency medical training. "Thanks, we'll let you know if we need you," she replied with obvious condescension.

After the attendant left, the lady passenger sitting next to me said, "Go on up! You can help more than the nurse that's there now."

I grabbed my Activator—a handheld device used by chiropractors to adjust the spine—and headed to the front of the coach section.

An elderly woman, sitting in a left-aisle seat and gasping for breath, held a set of dentures in her hand to allow more room through her air passage. She looked quite fragile and *very* scared. A nurse squatted in the aisle while measuring blood pressure and asking her questions about the medications in her purse.

I bent over the lady, who was white-as-a-sheet and obviously exhausted, looked into her eyes, and asked with careful enunciation, "W-h-a-t i-s y-o-u-r n-a-m-e, D-e-a-r?"

"Emma," she murmured.

Speaking softly, I asked her to take a deep breath and then tell me about her day.

"I was just released from the hospital this morning where I had my heart checked. I'm on my way to Seattle to live with my son because my granddaughter—who *had* been my caregiver—has deserted me. My heart is absolutely broken," she whimpered. The poor thing looked even more frail and frightened as she uttered these last words.

I asked Emma to lean forward in her seat so that I could place my hand on her neck and back and gently feel the condition of her spine. As I did so, I noted that her neck and upper back felt like a jumble of bones that had no place to call home. At that point, I asked if she had had any accidents recently.

"Yes, I fell down a few days ago and hurt my back and neck," she said.

As we talked, I noticed that her breathing was shallow and labored. "Emma, I'm going to adjust your neck so you can breathe normally; your body's life force will return."

She looked up at me with total confidence and understanding of exactly what I was saying and doing. The adjustment was quick and painless as Emma's bones moved into their proper alignment.

Immediately after I adjusted her spine, Emma was able to breathe normally. The flight attendant, who had observed us, was astounded, "She looks *so* much better! Look how she's brightening up. Her color is returning and her eyes don't look so vacant."

Emma leaned back into her seat and heaved a deep sigh. She then closed her eyes and relaxed for the first time since I had begun working with her.

I turned and asked the flight attendant if they had a banana—they're *loaded* with electrolytes—in the galley for Emma. No luck. "Do you have some room temperature water?" Again, no luck.

"We have *cold* water," a suddenly-perky flight attendant replied in a sincere attempt to be helpful.

"No, that will shock her system," I replied. "She's dehydrated; she needs electrolytes and tepid water ASAP! At the very least, lay her down so she can rest until we land."

Despite my suggestions, the nurse and flight attendant continued fussing over Emma, asking the same questions, taking and re-taking her blood pressure, and persistently resisting the idea that Emma was back to normal and just needed some warm water, a banana, and rest.

Finally, two flight attendants laid Emma across three vacant seats and let her rest. As soon as we landed, paramedics boarded the plane and began checking Emma's vital signs. After a few minutes, the senior paramedic stood and said, "This lady needs fluids and electrolytes. She's severely dehydrated." In vain, I waited for him to ask the banana question; he never did!

I walked back to my seat and began gathering my bags. The lady who had been sitting next to me and had encouraged me to go up front was still in her seat. She asked, "What did you do?"

"I adjusted her spine; that released her nervous system so it could do its own healing," I replied. When my seatmate nodded approvingly, I asked, "Are you familiar with Chiropractic?"

"Well, I *used* to be a nurse; and *now* I'm a flight attendant for this airline."

"Oh," I said. "Why didn't *you* go up front and help?"

"She didn't need *me*," my seatmate replied, "she needed *you!*"

As I walked toward the exit door, I silently blessed the Gift of Chiropractic and the power of the human body and spirit to heal itself—especially when interference is removed. As I moved past Emma, she looked up into my eyes, smiled a toothless grin, and gave me a frail thumbs-up!

Carol LeBlanc, DC
and
Vicki McConnell
LeBlanc Chiropractic
Costa Mesa, California

Horrors: Begone!

Charles B. Griffith was a prolific screenwriter and director best known for creating the screenplay for the 1960 cult classic, "The Little Shop of Horrors." By the time he was in his 70s, he had suffered excruciating, deep pain in his right femur for years. Walking was a major chore for this gentleman. In 2001, when the following poem was written, he was living in Ensenada, Mexico. He complained so much about his pain that a friend for whom I had been providing Chiropractic care decided to do something about it. Mr. Griffith's friend brought him to my office in Los Angeles, housed him in a hotel for eight weeks, and paid for his treatment.

When I released Mr. Griffith to return to Ensenada, the author gave me his cane. The following poem is the testimonial he sent to me after his return to Mexico:

Ptestimonial for Dr. Ptak*

I took the pain to my HMO.
  They said: "Take two Tylenol and call us next year."

I took it to my orthopedist.
  He offered me two new hips for the price of one.

I took it to my podiatrist.
  He trimmed my nails and gave me the boot.

I took it to my neurologist.
  He just got on my nerves.

I took it to my dermatologist.
  He skinned me, but it didn 't go away.

I took it to my herbalist.
  He handed me an acorn and said, "Eat this."

I took it to my acupuncturist.
  He stuck me for a couple of hundred.

I took it to my psychiatrist.
  He said it wasn't in my leg, it was in my head.

I took it to my proctologist.
  He just gave me a pain in the butt.

I took it to my paleotantric faith healer.
  He didn't believe me.

I finally took it to Dr. Ptak
  Who hooked me up to his leatherette rack,

And just when I thought my bones would crack,
  He took away the years of pain.

And...just for good measure
  He took away my cane.

                                    C. B. Griffith

In 2007, at the age of 77, Mr. Griffith passed away in San Diego of a heart attack. He left the world a rich legacy of humor for which he will long be remembered. His cane is still on display in my office, and the sight of it never fails to make me smile.

                                    Jeffrey Ptak, DC
                                    Ptak Wellness
                                    Los Angeles, California

* No folks, that's not a typo; the title, "Ptestimonial to Dr. Ptak," is just another example of Charles Byron Griffith's sense of whimsy.

14

A Chiropractic Menagerie

"We can judge the heart of a man by his treatment of animals."

Immanuel Kant
German Philosopher
(1724-1804)

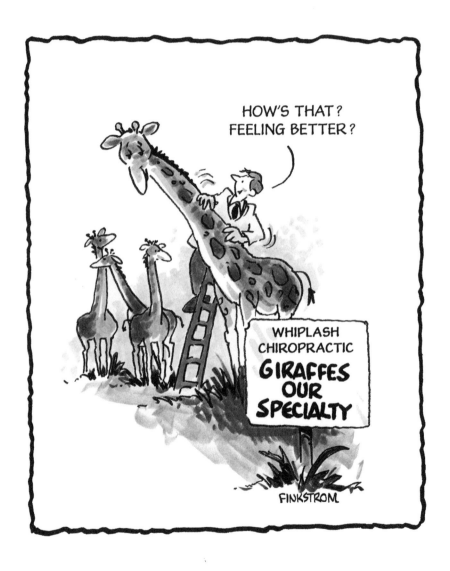

Reprinted by arrangement with Finkstrom Licensing International

A Life-or-Death Adjustment

"If there are no dogs in Heaven, then when I die I want to go where they went."

Will Rogers
Caring member of the human race
American, Cherokee Indian
Cowboy, star of 71 movies, friend of Presidents
His credo: "I never met a man I didn't like."
(1897-1935)

It is a fact—well-documented in healthcare journals—that companion animals can have a profound, positive effect on the psychological and physiological health of their owners. In recognition of this, the Parker College of Chiropractic in Dallas, Texas, offers its post-graduate Animal Chiropractic Program. This is currently the only such collegiate-based program in the world. It is my privilege to serve as the director of this program, to be on the faculty of this fine, caring, academic institution, and to operate the independent, campus-based, Parker Animal Wellness Clinic.

Some years ago, toward the end of a long day of seeing companion animal patients, I walked into an exam room to find a case that no veterinarian likes to see. It was a three-year-old poodle named FiFi that was paralyzed from the waist down. The pup's owner told me she had taken FiFi to her regular veterinarian a couple of days earlier. He said that her dog had a hurt back and needed immediate surgery or would never walk again. If she couldn't afford surgery, then the animal would have to be put to sleep.

The concerned owner was not a person of financial means and couldn't afford the surgery, so she took her dog back home in the hope it might get better on its own. Unfortunately, FiFi showed no signs of recovery. In fact, she was getting depressed because she couldn't walk and suffered the messy indignity of lost bladder and bowel control.

The dog's owner had spoken to a friend who told her about me and the Parker Animal Wellness Clinic. The friend recommended that she bring her dog to see me. My exam revealed that FiFi had a herniated disc in her lower spine. The bad thing was that I couldn't elicit a pain response in FiFi's rear legs. The absence of deep pain is a grave sign in these types of cases. Without surgery in the first twenty-four hours, almost none of these dogs ever walk again. I informed the owner of the very poor prognosis. I also told her I'd adjust FiFi and that we would simply have to hope for the best. I explained that if there was no improvement in one week to return to the clinic and I'd put FiFi to sleep.

It is a tremendous responsibility to treat *any* of God's creatures. This is especially true when you know that if you're not able to help them, they'll be put to sleep. I was in the position of literally making a life-or-death adjustment! So, I did some spinal traction work on FiFi and then gently gave her a Chiropractic adjustment. I recommended some supplements that the owner could start her on and told her to bring FiFi back to me the following Friday. I figured I would be seeing FiFi on that Friday for her "final" vet visit.

The next week went by as most weeks do—full of all sorts of busyness. To be honest, I completely forgot about FiFi. Then, Friday rolled around. Just before we were scheduled to close, in walked FiFi and her human companion! Yes, I said, "*in walked FiFi!*" Granted, her gait wasn't perfect, but she was *walking*. I picked her up, gave her a hug, and sat her on my exam table. I found that while she still had neurological problems, she was enormously improved. She could stand, she knew where her rear feet were, and she could feel it when I pinched her toes.

The owner told me that the afternoon after I had adjusted FiFi, the dog had gone home and slept the next twenty-four hours! The following morning, FiFi was whimpering to go outside to "do her duty." The owner followed my instructions, carried the dog out, and sat her in the grass. She told me that FiFi pulled herself up and, although very wobbly, stood to go to the bathroom and then lay back down. Throughout the week, FiFi got progressively stronger and stronger so that by Tuesday she started taking her first steps. By Friday, she was ambulating pretty well.

I adjusted FiFi again that day and saw her once-a-week for the next four weeks until I could finally say she was completely back to normal. It was nothing short of a miracle; and—had I not seen it with my own eyes—I'm not sure I would have believed it.

Clinically, there was no hope for this patient; and certainly, as a traditionally-trained veterinarian, I had very little to offer the animal other than surgery. Fortunately for me, and all of my patients, my life took an unusual twist almost thirty years ago when I was hired to teach anatomy at a new Chiropractic College in Dallas. At that time, I knew nothing about Chiropractic, but I *did* know how to teach. After seeing many human patients helped with Chiropractic care at the college, I wanted to learn this art so I could help my animal patients.

As a faculty member, I took some human Chiropractic classes and extrapolated what I learned back to my animal patients. A whole new world opened up for me *and* my patients. I still had a lot to learn; so I took additional coursework and passed the rigorous examination offered by the American Veterinary Chiropractic Association to become certified in Animal Chiropractic. My practice now is about eighty-percent Chiropractic care and twenty-percent traditional veterinary medicine. Had I not known about Chiropractic and how to adjust my patients, I'm convinced that FiFi would never have walked again and would certainly have been put to sleep.

Since starting at Parker, I've witnessed many similar cases with near-miracle results thanks to Chiropractic care. I'll always remember FiFi though, because she was such a severe case. I still see her for routine veterinary care and, as her owner calls them, "tune ups." I occasionally have to remind FiFi though, what I did for her years ago, because she's gotten a little grouchy in her old age. She even tried to bite me the last time I saw her. Now, *that's* appreciation for you!

Gene F. Giggleman, DVM
Animal Wellness Clinic
Parker College of Chiropractic
Dallas, Texas

The Cat Who Ate My Patient

I was tapping on my keyboard one morning when a small blur appeared at the edge of my vision.

"What the...?" I went outside to investigate and soon found a tiny bird at my feet. It had crashed into the window. The poor thing must have thought the reflection from the trees was the real thing. Blame Windex!

A few years earlier, Dr. Arno Burnier* and I had found a bird in just such a condition. "Zees happens all zee time at my house, Tedd," he said. (Imagine a French accent.) At the time, Arno lived in a house with *lots* of large windows.

"What do you do with them, Arno?"

"If I get zem in time, I can save zem. I just bring zee leetle neck to tension and give a tiny pull. *Voila!* You hear zee noise; they fly away soon." He demonstrated on the bird we had just found. It died. "We got eet too late," he said.[†]

Arno's words came back to me as I saw the tiny body on my doorstep. I gently picked up the bird. It was warm. It wasn't moving, but its eyes were open. I held his head by the occipital bone (the base of the skull), held the body firmly, brought it to tension, and "pop, pop, pop." I got some releases. "Wow, this is great," I thought. I put the bird down on the cold stoop and he started to flutter around. I ran into the house to get a shoebox as a "recovery room."

"I wonder if he has insurance," I thought. Ha! Ha!

Thirty seconds later; I was back. The bird was gone. He flew away. Full of self-congratulations, I thought, "I'll have to tell Arno about this."

Then I saw it. The bird was about 10 feet away, gently held in the mouth of our cat! I went nuts! The ground was muddy from a couple of days of rain, and I was wearing brand new white gym socks. To heck with the socks! I ran out to save my patient. The cat started loping away. I started screaming at him.

"You lousy piece of #@&%!" (Hey, I'm from Brooklyn.) "Gimme back my patient!"

Okay, it wasn't my finest moment. I'm not sure what the neighbors thought...but they shouldn't be snooping anyway.

I chased that darn cat around the property; but four legs beat two any day of the week. (I was a much better runner before evolution.) Anyway, the cat ran under the back deck with bird feathers sprouting from his mouth. I turned away in impotent rage. The cat ate my patient.

*Arno is a personal friend and internationally-renowned Chiropractic lecturer and retreat leader.

†In fairness to Arno, he has a pretty good record of saving birds. In fact, he sent me a picture of the last bird he saved at one of his retreats. Although it wasn't a paying registrant, he worked on it nevertheless, and it flew away.

Tedd Koren, DC
Founder and President
Koren Publications, Inc.
Hatfield, Pennsylvania

White Dandelion Puffs

"Animals are such agreeable friends—they ask no questions, they pass no criticisms."

George Eliot
Pen name for Mary Anne Evans
English author of *Silas Marner* and six other novels
(1819-1880)

It seemed like any normal summer day on our 120-acre farm in the middle of Wisconsin. The hay fields had recently been cut and the air smelled sweet and grassy. Our herd of fourteen alpacas was grazing in the pasture. Two baby alpacas, called crias, had been born a couple of weeks earlier and were jumping through the tall grass. When they first encountered a patch of gone-to-seed dandelions, they were startled by the white plumes of dandelion spray. Their surprise quickly turned to delight as they started *stomping* on the plants in order to see more puffs of white.

Sabrina was our last alpaca due to give birth that year; this would be her first baby. I checked on her, and she looked good. I figured it would probably be another week or two before we'd see her cria. With that, I felt comfortable leaving the farm to run errands. Understand, as a certified Animal Chiropractor, I'm an old pro at the alpaca-birthing process. Besides, Mother Nature always takes care of everything; I had absolutely nothing to worry about!

Alpacas have their babies during the day—late mornings to early afternoons—*waaaaay* easier than horses! When I returned to the farm, I noticed the alpacas were all together in the center of the pasture. Maybe Sabrina had had her baby early. Alpacas are such *wonderful* herd animals with strong group dynamics. After a cria is born, all of the other herd members visit to make its acquaintance. The first time I saw the herd that afternoon, I thought of *The Lion King* and "The True Circle of Life."

Walking through the pasture gate, I got my first inkling that something wasn't quite right. The other alpacas weren't calm; they were milling about...restless. And they were humming nervously. At first, I thought there might be a stray cat nosing around which meant the girls would chase him out of the pasture. After taking a few steps, though, I realized they weren't chasing *anything!*

Alarm bells rang in my head...I gasped...and started to jog.

"Easy girls, easy...," I said over and over as I worked my way inside the herd. Then I saw her. Sabrina was lying on her side— covered in bright, red blood. She seemed quite edgy, as though she didn't know what to do. Her legs made a sort-of "fence" that provided a low, protective barrier around her cria. My stomach clenched at the sight of so much blood. I stood there unsure of what to do. Our oldest alpaca touched me with her soft nose and stared into my eyes as if to say, "We're counting on you."

I picked up the limp, bloody cria and carried her out of the pasture toward the barn. The entire herd crowded around me, and I was thankful for their supportive presence. When I got to the double-Dutch barn doors, all the girls wanted to come inside with me. I wound up doing a glorified "chicken dance" to let myself, Sabrina, and her cria *inside* while keeping everybody else *outside*. It looked like a scene from a Disney movie with the heads of the rest of the herd poking in over the double-width Dutch door shelf. What's more, all of the girls were humming, "Hummmmmmm, hummmmmmmmmm." Given the circumstances, I concluded that this was female alpaca-talk for "What's going on? We want to help."

I dried the cria with a soft towel and disinfected her umbilical cord with iodine before setting her down on fresh straw in one of the stalls. Those were the easy things to do...the normal things.

Unfortunately, there was *nothing* normal about *this* cria. She was limp; something seemed majorly wrong with her legs. "Get up baby," I thought, "you need to nurse." Well, willpower wasn't working, so I decided to hold her up—all twenty-pounds of her—so she could nurse. This wasn't as easy as you'd think because it was all new to Sabrina. As I squatted next to the standing, first-time mother, she looked at me like, "You're gonna' touch me *where? I don't think so!*"

After several unsuccessful attempts, I managed to get Sabrina into a corner of the stall and hold her baby up. Oh, no! Not only couldn't the cria *stand*, she couldn't *hold her head up* either. "Okay," I thought, "Deep breath! Don't panic!" I held her tiny head up to the teat. She couldn't suck. She didn't even try to latch on. "*Colostrum,* this cria needs *colostrum!*" was my only thought. I knew full well that if this cria didn't get colostrum—thick milk loaded with vital, life-sustaining nutrients and anti-bodies only available from an alpaca mother for a short time after birthing—we'd have to subject her to a blood plasma trans-fusion within eight hours.

My body was coursing with adrenaline; and it took me a moment to realize what I was feeling. I gently stroked the cria's neck. Her atlas—the vertebra at the top of her spine—was sub-luxated! What a relief! In all of the panic and turmoil of wondering what to do for this cria, I finally realized there was something I *could* do. *I adjusted her neck!* Instantly, her sucking reflex kicked in. "Okay, baby girl, let's put that to use," I thought as I held her up to her mother's teat. "Hurray! She's nursing!" While she couldn't stand yet, at least she could nurse. After several minutes, I laid her down on the straw to rest while I peeled off my bloody, sweaty clothes.

An hour later, the cria was still unable to stand, but she was holding her head up. I decided it was time to check her pelvis. Sure enough, she had pelvic and sacral problems, so I adjusted those and then lifted her to nurse again.

Later that day, I was rewarded to see the most amazing thing: my baby cria was standing and nursing...*on her own!*

After her Chiropractic-assisted debut, it was less than a couple of weeks before our newly-named Sadie was jumping in the tall grass...and making white dandelion puffs with her fellow crias.

Cindy Conway, DC
Freedom Farm Chiropractic
Athens, Wisconsin

Dr. Conway is the author of
Essential Lies, a novel

She Was a One-Eyed Possum with a Crooked Smile

Hot Lips: the circumstances surrounding my first meeting with her were most unusual—and well worth an explanation. You see, I'm a physician and often need to be at the hospital into the late hours of the evening. When I finally got away that night, I faced the usual drive home. As I rounded a curve, I noticed an animal sitting in the middle of the road. I would later name this full-grown adult female opossum "Hot Lips."

I swerved to miss her; and as I passed, I noticed she didn't move. Knowing that something must be wrong, I pulled over, stopped the car, got out, and walked back to where she remained in a sitting position on the center line. It was dark; but I could faintly see blood coming from her mouth and hear the gurgle of blood down her throat. I suspected she had just been hit by another vehicle. After assessing that her body seemed free of injuries, I picked her up and gently placed her in the back of my car.

Most people are horrified to hear that I picked up a wild opossum on the road, but I was unafraid. You see, I had handled opossums before. I had raised several litters of orphaned opossums until they were mature enough to be released into the wild. I had handled and cared for injured adult opossums, too. Despite their gnarly appearance when frightened, I've found opossums to be among the sweetest, most gentle creatures on earth. Their wicked facial expressions and evil growls are all a façade to scare away threatening predators.

Opossums never get rabies, are resistant to snake venom, and can feign death when attacked. Their hands and feet are not unlike human hands and feet, and they usually like to grasp one of your fingers or your necklace when being held. Their fur is soft, and their tails are prehensile. Although they're considered to be a mean, rabid, filthy, worthless animal by most, the truth is that they are fascinating creatures, made perfectly by the hands of God, and a valuable part of our ecosystem.

Hot Lips was taken to my veterinarians, Drs. Donnie and Dawn DeLong, early the next morning. She had suffered mainly head and facial trauma. Examination and x-rays revealed a broken upper jaw and a shattered lower jaw. Both jaws had to be wired together to ensure proper healing. She also suffered fractured facial bones, a ruptured eardrum, and a right-eye injury requiring that her eye be removed. For the next week, I visited my little Hot Lips every day. I enjoyed holding and loving on her, and she enjoyed the foot massages I gave that always made her fall asleep.

After a week at the animal hospital, Hot Lips came home with me where she would finally heal. Even though her injuries healed well, she appeared to suffer from neck pain and muscle spasms. She constantly turned her head to one side to stretch the neck muscles on the opposite side. Despite my untrained massages and daily pain medicine, her neck problem worsened. It started affecting her quality of life, and I was desperate to find something that would help. I decided that Chiropractic care just might be the solution. At the risk of sounding absolutely absurd, I called my vet's office and asked for a referral. My suggestion was better received than expected, and soon I was given the name of Dr. Gina Carpenter, a human chiropractor with an interest in Animal Chiropractic.

Although Gina had never treated an opossum before, she immediately knew what the problem was. Observing that Hot

Lips' neck muscles were in spasm, Gina began treatment by applying traction to stretch them. This was followed by adjustments of the opossum's cervical (upper) spine to achieve correct alignment. Hot Lips responded quickly and profoundly to Gina's home visits. In no time, the head turning normalized and the pain obviously abated. Gina continued weekly home visits to adjust Hot Lips for the remainder of my precious and beloved opossum's life.

Although Hot Lips was a mere opossum, she was also a great deal more. Her gift, which she bestowed freely, was to make people smile and laugh. Often, I would bring pictures of Hot Lips—dressed in doggy clothes—to the hospital. Her pictures never failed to lift the spirits of my sick, and at times terminal, patients and their families. She touched the lives of many, and she brought four doctors together—an MD, two DVMs, and one DC. She was the catalyst for a deep and abiding friendship between our three families. I will always love, and forever be indebted to, my sweet Hot Lips.

Susan W. Grey, MD
Pulmonary and Critical Care Medicine
Conyers, Georgia

Donnie E. DeLong, DVM
and
Dawn D. DeLong, DVM
Animal Medical Center of Monroe
Monroe, Georgia

Gina B. Carpenter, DC
Complete Chiropractic
Snellville, Georgia

Our "Endeering" Experience

My husband, Tom, and I always knew we wanted a large family and the opportunity to be close with our children as they grew up. When deciding on a place to open our Chiropractic practice, we decided on a home office setting to achieve this family-raising goal. When choosing this home, it was important for us to be in a relatively busy community, and yet also to be as close to nature as possible. When we found our large home with a creek in the back and bordering a state park, we knew it was the perfect place.

Over the years, we encountered much wildlife. In the mornings, the feathered residents in our neighboring trees provided us with songbird symphonies. We encountered numerous forms of wildlife and—with the passage of time—raised abandoned raccoons, possum, birds, and bunnies along with the usual cats and dogs.

One of our most profound rescue experiences occurred late one summer afternoon. Our Labrador was barking furiously at the edge of the property. She was usually a quiet dog and only brought attention to herself when there was something very unusual happening. We followed her barking call and, to our absolute surprise, found her hovering over a young buck that was lying on the ground. Obviously petrified with fear, the buck made no attempt to move. At first, we thought he'd been hit by a car and had sustained a broken bone or other internal injury.

In any case, he needed help; and I knew if he was left out for the night, he might be harassed by foxes. I called over to my husband and insisted that we bring the buck closer to our home for protection. Using the tractor and a pallet, we dragged the heavy deer closer to the back porch. He appeared to be completely paralyzed with no ability to move. We settled him in for the night and I called a friend of ours whose specialty was animal rescue. She told us that he probably had "tick fever" and that every tick would have to be removed. After that, she continued, we'd need to get the deer drinking and eating again. My husband brushed the deer for at least an hour, pulling off hundreds of ticks. He filled a large bottle with water and siphoned it into the deer's mouth as the animal was unable to even lift his head. Some water seemed to be swallowed.

The next day, we continued to hydrate the deer; however he was still too weak to chew any food. Since both of us are chiropractors and know the power of an adjustment, we began to work on the buck's spine, particularly the neck area. Over the years, I had adjusted cats, dogs, horses, rabbits, squirrels, raccoons, possum...well, just about any mammal that came our way.

Every day, we gave the deer more water and checked his spine. After a couple of days, he began to eat, slowly-but-steadily. In the evenings, my husband would get next to him and lift him up from under his belly, encouraging him to stand. Slowly, the buck gained strength from much-needed nourishment, turning on the life force with adjustments, and a whole lot of passionate love from the entire family.

On the evening of the seventh day, Tom was performing his daily ritual of lifting the buck and helping him to steady and balance his weight. This time, the buck remained standing! Tom stepped back a bit, and the buck began delicate-but-sure steps toward the lawn. Thrilled at seeing these accomplishments, Tom ran into the house calling all six children and myself. We watched in awe...the buck was walking, step-by-step, toward the lawn. Someone brought out the video camera and Tom stood in front of the deer while filming his progress. He would step backwards and the deer would take careful steps toward him.

I remember it was a bit of a cloudy night. It had just stopped raining, but the clouds were still blocking the full moon. Tom continued to step backward, with the deer advancing toward him. With each step, the deer was more surefooted and strengthened. They got well onto the lawn when Tom looked the deer in the eyes and said, "You're free to go now." But the deer remained directly in front of him, not wavering from Tom's gaze. "What?" my husband asked; and he held out his free hand toward the deer. The deer stopped in stillness, looked right into Tom's eyes, and licked his hand as if to say, "Thank you...for nourishing me, for turning on my life force, and for loving me."

After he licked Tom's hand, the deer walked off in the direction of the woods, steady and free. Well, I think all eight of us were sobbing. The full moon broke through the parting clouds and we stood riveted and quite speechless watching the magnificent buck return to his home in the woods.

Within all life, there is an innate intelligence that is striving to express itself. Through this intelligence, we are all connected within a matrix of living, loving interaction. When this intelligence is nourished and nurtured, there is no telling its amazing ability to heal and express.

Jeanne Ohm, DC
Ohm Family Chiropractic
Media and Philadelphia, Pennsylvania

Dr. Ohm is the editor of
Pathways to Family Wellness
A magazine for new parents
Published by the
International Chiropractic Pediatric Association

Celebrate the Sky

I had not expected her to be so *big!*

Nor could I have guessed that, upon first sight, she would fill my heart with fear and awe...all in the same moment.

Truth be told, I'd never expected that I would *ever* treat a bird of prey.

One summer morning in 1998, I arrived at the veterinary clinic where—for nearly a decade—I had specialized in Animal Chiropractic. Entering the lab area, I was greeted by my long-time veterinarian friend, Dr. Maria.

"Would you mind looking at a hawk today, Dr. Julie?"

"A hawk? *Really*, are you serious?"

"Yes, we sometimes do *pro bono* work for the wildlife reha-bilitators. They've brought us a female hawk that was seriously injured when she flew into a plate-glass window. The hawk was found nearly dead, and someone called the rehab center to rescue her."

"Oh, no! *Of course* I'll help...if I can. How bad is she? Any fractures? Is she able to fly?"

"Well no, that's it. We've done everything we can to help her recover: acute care, radiographs, physical therapy...and the rehabilitator is one of the best at treating and handling birds of prey. She's excellent. But now, we're at a dead end. If the hawk can't fly, it's over."

"Do you believe that Chiropractic can help her, Maria?"

"We're out of options; I certainly hope so."

"So, how big *is* this bird of prey?"

"She's two-feet long, and her wingspan is over four feet!"

"Wow!" I exclaimed, more than a little intimidated.

"The problem is that after all we've done, this bird still can't fly because her head is rotated to the right side and stuck there."

Maria reached for a book on avian anatomy and opened to a skeletal diagram of *Accipiter gentilis*—the Northern Goshawk.

"Stuck to the right? But no fractures?" I cringed as I looked at the diagram revealing fragile, porous bones honeycombed with air pockets designed for facile flight. It was dawning on me how dangerous this could be. Not just dangerous for *me* in handling a full-sized hawk, but dangerous for *the hawk* as well. If she suddenly turned her head during my adjustment, or if one of us jerked reflexively during the procedure, my fingers might fracture her neck and kill her instantly!

"So, what if I can't help her?"

"That's just it. Your treatments will either allow the rehabilitator to set her free…. Or she'll spend the rest of her life in a cage at the rehab center. She could live another sixteen years or more!"

I composed myself, gathered my files, and entered the exam room. Barbara, a tall, proud woman, stood over a large dog crate in the center of the exam table. I extended my hand, "Hello, I'm Dr. Kaufman."

Barbara studied me with calculating eyes. She did not extend her hand to meet mine. "Birds are very sensitive to movement," she warned. Her voice was strong and calm. "You'll have to move slowly and carefully. Her talons are razor sharp." She watched my reaction, our eyes locking. "Her beak can tear flesh from bone in a split second." Barbara was dead serious.

"How would you like to proceed?" I asked.

"I'll handle her for you. The doctor told you about the injury?" I nodded.

"Do *everything* you can," Barbara said with firm urgency. She paused before continuing…softly this time, "Thank you."

I stood motionless as Barbara slipped her right hand—clad in an extremely-thick, elbow-length leather glove—into the crate and skillfully extracted the enormous bird. As the hawk's red eye with its piercing black pupil studied me—just as Barbara had done previously, I deliberately slowed my breathing to present as calm and fear-free a demeanor as possible.

The hawk's head was bent oddly to the right, and her right shoulder was noticeably higher as a result of her injury. As an Animal Chiropractor, I'm sensitized to immediately pick up imbalance, out-of-sync lines of the body, muscles bulging taut under fur and feather, and structural integrity misaligned by injury. Immediately, I could see her distress; her lower cervical spine arched unnaturally, her shoulder and upper back hunching where her body had absorbed the trauma of the impact.

Barbara then produced a soft, small leather hood. "This will cover her eyes and keep her calm. If she senses movement, she could panic and slice one of us with her talons." Barbara gently slipped the hood over the hawk's head, covering its eyes, secured it, and then nodded that she was ready.

"I can help her," I said quietly, reaching gently toward the hawk's back with steady, soft hands. My fear evaporated as I tuned in to the hawk's body. It was a beautiful honor to touch her, to be a part of this healing and grace.

My hands began communicating with her delicate skeletal structure, and initially discovered lower cervical misalignments. As I gently adjusted them, the hawk remained calm and receptive. Feeling increasingly relaxed, my breath slowed further and the external world ceased to exist. In a near-mystical way, my total consciousness focused on the healing process. I gently slid one hand under the hawk's right wing and palpated her shoulder. There, I found and corrected several subluxations in her neck, wing, and back. The hawk continued to remain calm and slowly turned her neck to the left as the subluxations were released.

"I see that she can move her neck much better already," Barbara observed, approvingly. "She's calm." She removed the hood and the magnificent bird once again turned her left eye to me.

Seeing the hawk without her hood, I felt a much deeper, wild connection that permeated my body. "She's amazing!" I exclaimed. I could still feel the warmth of the hawk's body tingling in my fingertips.

Barb brought the hawk to my office for three more treatments. On each occasion, the bird remained calm and receptive. Her range of motion steadily increased, and her ability to extend her wings improved greatly.

Shortly after the hawk's final adjustment, I received a note from Barb: "Appreciate you taking time to help our winged people. You are so special. We are planning to release the Goshawk next week. She'll fly back to her people."

Soon afterward, I got a call from Barb. Here is my "earwitness" account of her telephone report on the hawk's release:

"We drove her to the wildlife sanctuary at dawn where we would say our final words to our winged sister. My crew and I arrived at our release point before sun-up. We made sure she was well nourished the night before so she could have the best chance to adapt to her freedom after so many months. She was calm, much as she'd been in your office.

"We slid the crate from the back of the SUV, doing our final check as I eased her onto my gloved hand. There was no hood this time. I held her for several moments so she could explore the trees, the sun, and the sounds. She let out a loud screech and then there was silence.

"After a few moments, we heard the returning calls of other birds that we hoped were her own kind. She turned her head easily and began to spread her wings, stretching them fully. The sun was just rising and her fully-spread wings obscured the horizon. I pictured the tail of a Wright whale as she breeches the ocean surface to celebrate the sky.

"My hand lifted into the air as her enormous wings caught the gusting wind; I nearly lost her to the sky. But she folded her wings, calmed down, and rested again on my hand. I untied the leather leg band, the last remaining tether on her captivity.

"And in that final connection between woman and hawk, I thrust my arm high. The Goshawk spread her wings to an awesome, full-four-foot span and, for a moment, I could not see the sun for her magnificence. She rose up and down carrying my arm with her, pumping her wings, assessing her freedom. Her eye caught mine in the final moments before she married with sky and sunlight and her calling. Then she pushed with incredible force against my arm, propelling herself toward the sun.

"We cheered as we watched her touch the sky; our hearts filled with love, our eyes filled with tears. She was airborne...she was *free!*"

Julie Kaufman, DC
Animal Holistic Care Specialists of Wisconsin
Marshall, Wisconsin

Dr. Kaufman is the author of
Crossing the Rubicon:
Celebrating the Human-Animal Bond in Life and Death
and
JointYoga for Animals: Strength, Flexibility, Balance

Acknowledgments

Between the time the first story for *The Well-Adjusted Soul* was acquired and our Fall 2010 publication date, two full years will have elapsed. In that interval, a number of people made important contributions to this project. Your co-authors would like to take this opportunity to recognize those individuals.

More than 4,000 stories and testimonials were considered as possible candidates for our book. This group included stories solicited by Dr. LaMarche from his many friends and colleagues, submissions resulting from our Parker College of Chiropractic (PCC) Story Contest announcement e-blasted to more than 40,000 chiropractors in early 2010, patient testimonials and stories featured on thousands of Chiropractic websites, and interview-based stories solicited and written by Don Dible.

The 75 stories in this book were selected based on the efforts of our conscientious, dedicated Story Contest Judges (SCJs). They are, in alphabetical order: Katharine du Quesnay, DC; Steve Fonso, DC; Michael W. Hall, DC; William Charles Hollensed, DC; Heather Jones, DC; Steven King; Margaret Koski; Randy J. Koski, DC; Gilles A. LaMarche, DC; Jason P. Lamarche, DC; Daniel F. Lavanga, DC; DeAnn Mabry; Alexandra McKnight; Stacey Olson, DC; Catherine Quagliana; Fontaine K. Richardson, PhD; Eric G. Russell, DC; Jean-Marc Slak, DC; and Elizabeth Wiebe.

Several people were helpful in recommending authors who might be willing to write and submit a story for our contest. Individuals providing such referrals included: Leslie Means, Executive Director, Animal Veterinary Chiropractic Association; Jeanne Ohm, DC, Executive Director, International Chiropractic Pediatric Association; Angela Kargus, former Director, Public & Media Relations, American Chiropractic Association; and Gene Giggleman, DVM, Dean of Academic Affairs at PCC.

A special thank you goes to Lily Xu of Lily Xu Designs in Pleasanton, California, for her subtle cover graphic that singularly identifies the spine and nervous system as the focus of this book.

Randy Evert and Jack Lindstrom of Finkstrom Licensing International custom-created dozens of Chiropractic-themed cartoons from which 14 were chosen for inclusion in this book.

Henri Nuber, Publisher/CEO of *DC Products Review*, was most helpful in publicizing our Story Contest through an article in his magazine. Others that provided publicity included: D. John Bray, Public Relations Director, D'Youville College; Ricardo Fujikawa, DC, MD, Head of Studies-Chiropractic, RCU Escorial Maria Cristina, Madrid, Spain; Joel E. Margolies, DC, Publisher of the Chirosmart.net e-letter; and Angela Kargus, former Director, Public & Media Relations, American Chiropractic Association.

Among the many staff members at PCC deserving recognition for their contributions are Jesse Green, General Counsel for his expertise in reviewing and creating agreements; Dustin Dollar, Director of College Merchandising and Matt Eiserloh, Chief Marketing Director for their support in getting the book to print and making it available to the world; and Cheryl Moss, Executive Assistant to Dr. LaMarche for keeping all correspondence timely and accurate and being such a wonderful relationship builder.

In addition to the feedback Don Dible received from our 19 SCJs, he relied on a small circle of friends—many of whom are also professional writers—to provide editing feedback and commentary before submitting selected stories to our SCJs. This group included: Aina Barry, Scherry Cooley, the late Alice Dible, Pam and Ken Dougherty, Kathleen Hawkins, Calder Lowe, Midge Pierce, Peter Turla, Faye Whitman, and Robert and Betty Wroe.

Due to the size of this project, we may have overlooked the names of some people who contributed along the way. If so, we apologize; but please know that your efforts were helpful in bringing the message of Chiropractic's healing power to many thousands who might otherwise never have known about it.

Meet Fabrizio Mancini, DC

Dr. Fabrizio Mancini is an internationally-acclaimed bilingual speaker, author, educator, philanthropist, and president of one of the world's leading Chiropractic Colleges. His childhood dreams of serving humanity ignited in Texas where he pursued pre-medicine at the University of Dallas while preparing to become a neurosurgeon. It was there that he discovered his true passion in life—empowering individuals to take responsibility for their own health.

He enrolled as a student at Parker College of Chiropractic in 1987 recognizing the potential for preventing disease and educating patients in a wellness lifestyle. Upon graduation in 1993, he launched the Mancini Chiropractic Center in Dallas, Texas. In 1999, having been mentored by the late Chiropractic pioneer, Dr. James W. Parker, it was no surprise that Dr. Mancini was summoned to head Parker College. Today, he spends most of his time leading this institution to historic accomplishments in education, and professional and personal development seminars. Dr. Mancini travels the world inspiring thousands each year with his innovative messages of success, service, health, and wellness. But, when asked, he would say his favorite time is that spent with his lovely wife, Alicia, and their two sons, Gianni and Luciano.

Dr. Mancini's enthusiasm for life is contagious and has earned him acclaim including Humanitarian of the Year, Heroes for Humanity Award, Chiropractor of the Year, CEO Award, Vision Award, Crystal Apple Educators Award, ACA & TCA President's Award, induction into the Wellness Revolutionaries Hall of Fame, and more.

Dr. Mancini has given testimony before the White House Commission on Complimentary and Alternative Medicine and has served for many years on the Texas Governor's Advisory Council on Physical Fitness. He has authored numerous journal articles and has been featured in newspapers and magazines nationwide.

He is an active member of the National Speakers Association. He has been inducted as a Fellow of the International College of Chiropractors (FICC), the American College of Chiropractors (FACC), and the International Chiropractic Association (FICA).

Dr. Mancini co-authored *Chicken Soup for the Chiropractic Soul* with bestselling authors, Jack Canfield and Mark Victor Hansen. He has been a frequent guest of CNN Español with more than 38 million viewers. He received the honor of having Mexico's leading university, UNEVE, name its library after him.

Meet Gilles A. LaMarche, DC

Dr. Gilles LaMarche is a successful chiropractor, passionate healer, accomplished author, inspiring bilingual professional speaker, and certified personal development coach. Dr. LaMarche found his calling as a healer when, at the age of twelve, he was taken to a chiropractor after years spent as an "unwell" child. His only expectation was that a chiropractor might help him resume regular activities without pain; little did he know that this would change the course of his life. Discovering the science, art, and philosophy of Chiropractic led him to a vision for better health. This vision: to help the world discover the importance and value of taking personal responsibility for overall health and well-being naturally.

After completing a BS at the University of Toronto and a Doctor of Chiropractic degree at the Canadian Memorial Chiropractic College, he enjoyed sharing this philosophy with his patients in private practice in Northern Ontario from 1979-2004. During this period, he served on numerous volunteer boards including the College of Chiropractors of Ontario (CCO) whose mandate is to protect the public interest. He was honored to serve as president of the CCO for two years. In 2005, he was voted Canadian Chiropractor of the Year by readers of the *Canadian Chiropractor* magazine. He has spoken to audiences throughout Canada, the United States, Mexico, the Caribbean, Australia, Japan, Europe and Scandinavia.

Dr. LaMarche is the author and co-author of many books including *Chiropractic from the Heart*, *Steering Your Ship Called Life*, *Tired of Being Sick and Tired*, *Say Yes to Chiropractic Success*, and *The Parker System for Professional Success* (PSPS). A member of the Parker College postgraduate faculty since 1990, he has received numerous awards from this organization including Team Teacher of the Year and Mentor of the Year. In 2006, he became Director of Parker Seminars, and in 2008, accepted a VP position at Parker College of Chiropractic. Through Parker Seminars, Dr. LaMarche has continued to advance and unite the Chiropractic profession while encouraging people to take responsibility for the gift of health.

He believes in the great importance of commitment and responsibility to the world in which we live. He is a doctor, a teacher, a friend, and, most importantly: Dad to three terrific young adults. His mission is to help all those he meets achieve their full potential.

Meet Donald M. Dible, MS

On April 25, 2010, Alice M. Dible—Don's beloved wife of 42 years—passed away after a three-year battle with breast cancer. While the suffering is unimaginably dreadful for a terminally-ill cancer patient, a loving husband is not immune to the emotional toll it takes as he contemplates life without his soulmate.

It is generally accepted that hard work—doing something that provides deep psychological satisfaction—is effective therapy for dealing with grief. In Don's case, that's what service as editor of *The Well-Adjusted Soul* has provided—*therapy!* His path to writing began in an unusual way.

After graduating from MIT (BSEE) and Stanford University (MSEE), Don enjoyed a seven-year engineering career. With the end of the Cold War, aerospace fell on hard times and, in 1971, Don founded The Entrepreneur Press. He then self-published *Up Your OWN Organization! A Handbook for Entrepreneurs* with an Introduction by Robert Townsend, former Chairman of Avis-Rent-a-Car and author of what was—at the time—the #1 *New York Times* bestseller: *Up the Organization*. Two weeks after its publication, Don's book was adopted as a text at Stanford University. Then, the Wharton School followed suit as did more than 150 other academic institutions. In 1984, Don sold his publishing company to Prentice-Hall. To date, he has worked on more than 60 books including *Chicken Soup for the Dental Soul* (co-author) and *Chicken Soup for the Country Soul* (editor).

In the fall of 2008, Don was driving his wife home in the carpool lane of a six-lane-each-way California freeway from the Valley Cancer Institute in Los Angeles where she was an outpatient. Suddenly, the Dibles' Crown Victoria sustained a blowout, spun out of control, and hit a concrete wall almost head-on. Alice sustained no injuries, but Don experienced severe back spasms almost immediately. His internist prescribed x-rays, Vicodin, and Flexoril and told him to go to bed. Drugged out, Don awoke eighteen hours later—still in pain—and decided that narcotics and muscle relaxants were not for him.

The next day, he received his first Chiropractic adjustment from Dr. Cody Masek in Temecula, California, experienced almost immediate relief, and decided to create an anthology of Chiropractic stories. Soon after, he met Dr. Gilles LaMarche at the 2009 Parker Seminar in Las Vegas. The rest is history. Don is certain that—just as she did during their long marriage—Alice is now cheering him on...from Heaven.

You may contact Don at dondible@dmdhousebooks.com.

Meet Your Authors and Story Sponsors

Claudia Anrig, DC, a 1982 graduate of Life Chiropractic College, has been in full-time practice for the past 29 years and is the founder of the first comprehensive pediatric program and community outreach. She is the past president, and currently serves on the board, of the International Chiropractic Pediatric Association (www.icpa4kids.org) and is on the post-graduate faculty of several Chiropractic Colleges. Dr. Anrig's textbook, *Pediatric Chiropractic*, is the first of its kind and has been a breakthrough in helping chiropractors help children.

Susan Boerchers is a freelance writer based in Easton, Pennsylvania. Her articles have appeared in *The Family Digest, ParentGuide, Working Writer,* and *Leaders in Life Science.* She is currently at work on a novel.

Chris W. Burfield is the founder of the Chiropractic Secret Society, an online community that is dedicated to helping chiropractors serve more people and save more lives. Membership in the Chiropractic Secret Society is 100% FREE and available to Chiropractors only. To become a member, simply visit www.css1895.com. Chris shares life with his beautiful wife, Nicole, and their adorable daughter, Baleigh. The Burfield family currently resides in McKinney, Texas.

Arno Burnier, DC, a 1977 graduate of Sherman College of Chiropractic, is a powerful and charismatic speaker. A veteran of 20 years in practice, he is a renowned national and international lecturer on Health, Healing, Wellness, and Chiropractic. As a graduation speaker for Chiropractic Colleges and regular lecturer within Chiropractic forums, his message has transformed thousands of lives. His penetrating and powerful style, combined with heart, experience, insight, and simplicity, inspires audiences worldwide. He reaches into people's minds, hearts, and souls. He founded Master Piece Seminars, MLS Adjusting Seminars, Café of Life, and Zeechi. Contact info: 108 Latigo Road, Durango, CO 81301. P: 970.247.0004, E: arno@fone.net.

Brian O. Burns, DC, FICA, received his BS in 1979 from the University of Dayton and his DC from Life Chiropractic College in 1983. He has been in full-time family practice in Tampa Bay for 27 years. His youngest patient was two-minutes old and his oldest patient was 98-years old. He has a passion for sports, adjusts professional and varsity teams, and is a founding member of the Life University Rugby Team. He served on the Board of the Florida Chiropractic Society as their VP. He has also served as president of the PAC and as a Florida State representative to the International Chiropractic Association. He is a Fellow of the ICA. Dr. Burns is husband to GiGi and father of four. P: 813.935.8300, E: brianburnsdc@verizon.net.

Donna Cantalupo, DC, attended Dickinson College before earning her Doctor of Chiropractic degree in 1986 from National College of Chiropractic. She has been in private practice in her hometown of East Hanover, New Jersey, for the past 24 years. She continues to promote health and wellness in her community and adjusts local athletes. Dr. Cantalupo is past president of the East Hanover Board of Health. She enjoys spending time with her husband, Bill, and their three children, Alexis, Billy, and Taylor, who have been under Chiropractic care since birth.

Edward T. Caputo, DC, received his BS from Providence College in 1985 and his DC from National College of Chiropractic in 1990. He has been in private practice for almost two decades, serving his community with Chiropractic care. In his spare time, he enjoys being active in his children's athletic activities and coaches softball. He may be reached at Caputo Chiropractic, 1040 Oaklawn Avenue, Cranston, RI 02920. P: 401.944.2221, E: dred@caputochiropracticri.com.

Alan B. Carnathan, DC, graduated from Logan College of Chiropractic in Chesterfield, Missouri, in 1978. A chiropractor for more than 31 years, his rural practice has grown into a family wellness practice focusing on spine rehabilitation and acupuncture. Dr. Carnathan has incorporated acupuncture in his practice for more than 25 years, mentoring with numerous leaders in this field. President of Slack, Inc., he and his wife, Susan, designed and patented the Max-Relax® face cushion for clinical use. You may contact Dr. Carnathan at Carnathan Chiropractic Clinic, 5 Shiloh Road, Greers Ferry, AR 72067. P: 501.825.7200, E: carnathanclinic@sbcglobal.net.

Gerard W. Clum, DC, a 1973 Palmer College of Chiropractic graduate, has been a faculty member at his alma mater, a founding faculty member at Life Chiropractic College, and the first president of Life Chiropractic College West. He has served on the board of directors or as an officer of the Association of Chiropractic Colleges, the Council on Chiropractic Education, the International Chiropractors Association, the Foundation for Chiropractic Progress, and the World Federation of Chiropractic. As the most senior Chiropractic College administrator in the world, he began his 30th year as president in 2010. Dr. Clum has been acknowledged as Chiropractor of the Year by ICA, Man of the Year by *Dynamic Chiropractic*, and as one of the top five leaders of the Chiropractic profession in a *Dynamic Chiropractic* readers' poll.

Cindy Conway, DC, lives with her husband, cockatiel, cats, dog, horses, goats, llamas, and alpacas on a large farm in Wisconsin. She has been in practice since graduating from Logan College of Chiropractic in 1983. She is also a certified lifetime member of the American Veterinary Chiropractic Association. She has been published in the *Journal of Clinical Chiropractic Pediatrics* and has written a novel, *Essential Lies*. You can visit her at www.cindyconwaydc.com.

David Covey, DC, is a graduate of the Canadian Memorial Chiropractic College (CMCC) in Toronto. Teacher, public speaker, and clinician at a family-based wellness practice, he has a Bachelor of Science degree in Premedicine from Bob Jones University. Dr. Covey's love and passion is his family. God has blessed him with a beautiful wife, Faith-Anne, and three wonderful children, Hope, Grace, and Nathan. He may be contacted at New Freedom Chiropractic, 2016 Tenth Line

Road, Unit 7, Orleans, Ontario, Canada, K4A 4X4. P: 613.837.9777, F: 613.248.5162, E: info@findfreedom.ca, W: www.findfreedom.ca.

Jessica Crocker-Idone is the proud mother of three beautiful children. Two of her children faced great challenges ranging from seizures to chronic chest infections. In the midst of a fast-paced life filled with anxiety and fear, they lost hope. Then, a ray of hope began to shine through after meeting Dr. Covey from New Freedom Chiropractic. Almost three years later, under Chiropractic care, her family has been given the best gift of all—health. She devotes her life to enjoying her family and spreading the word of the benefits of Chiropractic care.

Renée Dallaire, DC, received her BS in nursing sciences from University Laval, Québec, in 1986 and her Doctorate of Chiropractic from the Palmer College of Chiropractic in 1991. The mother of two young adults, she lives by her mission: Every day through Chiropractic, I touch people that come my way. By the expression of my love, they feel enlightened, and they regenerate light to the end of time. Today, Dr. Dallaire practices in Pointe-Claire, a suburb of Montreal. Her beautiful professional office and service-oriented team attract patients of all ages. E: chiropratiquedessources@bellnet.ca, P: 514.630.1113, W: www.chiropratiquedessources.com.

John F. Demartini, DC, graduated with honors from Texas Chiropractic College in 1982, He is a chiropractor, human behavioral specialist, educator and international authority on healing and maximizing human awareness and potential. His studies have spanned numerous disciplines, and his teachings provide answers and solutions to many of life's questions and challenges. As a bestselling author and writer of over 40 published books, 160 manuscripts, and thousands of articles, Dr. Demartini is an educator who constantly travels the globe teaching students from all backgrounds and disciplines. Dr. Demartini is founder of the Demartini Institute, and originator of the Demartini Method. For more information on Dr. John Demartini and upcoming events contact The Demartini Institute, E: info@drdemartini.com, P: 713.850.1234, W: www.drdemartini.com.

Billy DeMoss, DC, is a 1985 graduate of the Los Angeles College of Chiropractic. He has practiced Chiropractic in Newport Beach, California, for 25 years. Dr. DeMoss started a philosophy group called the Dead Chiropractic Society to perpetuate the principles, history, and philosophy of Chiropractic. He also hosts an annual wellness and music festival called the California Jam that highlights the best speakers in Chiropractic and wellness. Dr. DeMoss can be contacted at P: 949.250.0600, E: dcs@deadchiropracticsociety.com, W: www.deadchiropracticsociety.com and www.caljam.org.

Joe Dispenza, BS, DC, earned his Doctor of Chiropractic degree from Life University and his BS degree with an emphasis in Neuroscience. His book, *Evolve Your Brain: The Science of Changing Your Mind*, connects the subjects of thought and consciousness with the brain, mind, and body. He is also featured in the award-winning film, *What the BLEEP Do We Know!?* When not traveling, writing, and lecturing, he is busy seeing patients at his Chiropractic clinic near Olympia, Washington. He may be contacted at Encephalon LLC, PO Box 772, Rainier, WA 98576; P: 360.446.3152, F: 360.446.3150; E: info@drjoedispenza.com; W: www.drjoedispenza.com and www.rainierchiro.com.

George B. Donnelly, DC, is a 1995 graduate of Life Chiropractic College in Marietta, Georgia. He is currently practicing Network Spinal Analysis with his wife, Lois Donnelly, DC. Their office is located at 6 Office Park Circle, Suite 203, Birmingham, AL 35223. To contact Drs. Donnelly please call 205.313.1792 or visit their website: TouchOfLightWellness.com.

Simon Floreani, DC, is a 1995 RMIT University graduate and leading Australian Doctor of Chiropractic. As President of the Chiropractors' Association of Australia and the first-ever chiropractor on the Board of Directors and Executive Committee of the Allied Health Professions-Australia—the peak body representing the third pillar of health—he leads Chiropractic to the forefront of health care delivery in Australia. With his acclaimed wife and bestselling author, Dr. Jennifer Barham-Floreani, he is CEO and co-founder of Vitality Organic Allied Health, a health and wellness community super-centre with seven DC associates in Melbourne. Dr. Floreani is a steering committee member of the Australian Federal Government Task Force on health reform and chronic disease management. He is also a highly sought-after media spokesperson on Allied Health-related issues across Australia.

Ryan French, DC, is a graduate of the Canadian Memorial Chiropractic College (CMCC) in Toronto. A health coach, teacher, and writer, he has earned a Degree in Kinesiology from McMaster University in Hamilton and is a post-doctorate Fellow of the International Chiropractic Pediatric Association. Dr. French shares life with his loving wife ,Suzanne, and their four children. He may be contacted at Inside Out Family Chiropractic, 27 King Street East, Bolton, Ontario L7E 1C2 Canada. P: 905.951.9911, F: 905.951.9231, E: info@insideoutchiro.org, W: www.insideoutchiro.org.

Martin Furlong, DC, is a second-generation chiropractor who has experienced natural health care exclusively his whole life. He is a 1986 graduate from Northwestern College of Chiropractic. Dr. Furlong has received advanced clinical training in Nutrition Response Testing. The primary goal of his clinic is to restore bodies through holistic care. You can contact Dr. Furlong at MetroEast Wellness Center in St. Paul, Minnesota. E: metroeastchiropractic@msn.com or P: 651.771.1703.

Carrie Ann Gallagher, DC, graduated with honors from Parker College of Chiropractic in 2004. Originally from Canada, she has moved to Melbourne, Australia, and has practiced at a family-based wellness practice since 2004. She is a natural-born communicator and educator. Dr. Gallagher has been published in *Pathways to Family Wellness*. She can be contacted at E: cagallagher@gmail.com, W: www.beingwellhealthcare.com.au.

Judith Gallagher, DC, is a graduate of the National College of Chiropractic in Illinois. She may be contacted at Caputo Chiropractic, 1040 Oaklawn Avenue, Cranston, RI 02920. P: 401.944.2221.

Gene Giggleman, DVM, is a *magna cum laude* graduate of Texas A & M Veterinary School where he was awarded the prestigious Cable Scholarship in small animal medicine. Dr. Giggleman is now Dean of Academic Affairs at Parker College. He has been awarded the Outstanding Teacher Award more than 30 times, a testament to his passion for teaching and his belief in his students. A practicing veterinarian who has been adjusting animals for more than 15 years, he has run several successful small animal veterinary practices in the DFW area since 1981. In spite of his busy schedule, Dr. Giggleman manages to find time to lecture around the country on both the fundamentals and benefits of Animal Chiropractic. He is currently serving as president of the American Veterinary Chiropractic Association.

Kent S. Greenawalt, President and CEO of Foot Levelers, Inc., has made a significant impact on the Chiropractic profession. In 2003, he led a group of individuals to form the Foundation for Chiropractic Progress (FCP). He currently serves as the Founder and Chairman of the FCP. In addition to his leadership at Foot Levelers, Kent is a committed supporter of Chiropractic education as evidenced by the numerous grants, research studies, donations, and scholarships awarded. W: www.footlevelers.com.

Susan W. Grey, MD, received her MD in 1990 from the Medical College of Georgia. After completing a three-year residency in Internal Medicine, she went on to finish a three-year fellowship in Pulmonary and Critical Care at the University of Tennessee. She retired in 2009 after fourteen years of practicing her subspecialty in Atlanta. Today, she shares her life and home with her husband, Jerry, thirteen dogs, four horses, a hedgehog, and a three-legged guinea pig. Animals have always been her utmost passion. She hopes to one day apply her knowledge of human medicine to advance the field of critical care in veterinary medicine. Susan can be reached at possumtrack@hotmail.com.

Michael W. Hall, DC, FIACN, a graduate of the Parker College of Chiropractic, is a renowned Chiropractic neurologist and educator. He has nearly two decades of experience in both teaching and clinical practice in the Dallas/Fort Worth area. He is also a popular public speaker about brain health and spinal wellness. For more information about Dr. Hall's practice, please visit wwww.hallchiropracticwellnesscenter.com or call 214.373.0002. E: mhall@parkercc.edu.

Bill Hannouche, BS, DC, has a Bachelor of Science Degree and an Honor Degree in Biology from York University in Toronto, Canada. He was accepted, but declined, admittance to Toronto School of Medicine once he discovered Chiropractic. Starting at Palmer College of Chiropractic, he finished at Sherman Chiropractic College. He taught at both Sherman and Life Colleges and has been a popular speaker on local radio and television for years. He has been in private practice for over 28 years and looks forward to his son, Nicholas, currently a Sherman student, joining him in the future. For more information about Dr. Hannouche's practice, please visit www.drhannouche.com or call 864.583.5649.

B. J. Hardick, DC, was named after the Developer of Chiropractic, B. J. Palmer, and was born into a passionate Chiropractic lifestyle. Dr. Hardick is a graduate of Life University and has now served the Chiropractic profession for more than 20 years. Practicing in London, Ontario, Canada, Dr. Hardick serves patients in the facility originally established by his father in 1971. He runs a subluxation-centered family practice and extends his message through his own seminars, teaching the principles for living that he has championed his entire life. Dr. Hardick is co-author of the bestselling *Maximized Living Nutrition Plans* used in clinics worldwide. W: www.DrHardick.com.

Andrew P. Hatch, DC, is a 1993 graduate of Parker College of Chiropractic in Dallas, Texas. He is Vice Chair on the Board of Trustees of Parker College where he has served since 2005. Dr. Hatch has resided and practiced in Lisbon, Portugal, since 1994 and was the fifth chiropractor in the country. He is the owner of several successful clinics in and around the Lisbon area. He is a co-founder of the Portuguese Chiropractors Association, APQ, and served as Vice President and Secretary for several years working actively toward regulation. Dr. Hatch is also an active public speaker, practice consultant, and coach. He is currently expanding his company GWC, Global Wellness Corporate, to provide in-house Chiropractic services and wellness consulting to large corporations throughout Europe.

Donald G. Hattier, D.C. graduated from National College of Chiropractic in 1985 and then moved to Bethany Beach, Delaware, to begin his Chiropractic practice. Now, nearly 25 years later, he has built that practice into a thriving multi-service Chiropractic center, complete with family medicine, podiatry, and more. Along with his dedication to Chiropractic, Dr. Hattier has always shown a strong commitment toward community. He hosts a bi-weekly radio talk-show educating local residents about Chiropractic and also serves as an elected official on his local school board. For those needing Chiropractic care while vacationing at the Delaware beaches, Dr. Hattier can be reached at 302.539.7063.

Laura S. Hattier graduated from Salisbury University in 1988. From that point on, she has been busy helping her husband run his Chiropractic office as well as raising their family of four gifted and accomplished children. In addition to caring for the Hattier home and business, Laura has demonstrated an active interest in matters of faith. For nearly 20 years, she's been teaching and preaching in a variety of church settings and has been published in several of her area's regional newspapers. Currently, she authors a weekly faith column for Gannett publications.

William Charles Hollensed, DC, graduated from Lincoln Chiropractic College in 1970. He has refocused from private practice to full-time ministry as the President of the Christian Chiropractors Association. He has had the joy of providing Chiropractic care on numerous short-term mission trips. He has been blessed to be married to his bride, Lorna, for 42 years. He can be contacted at 630.202.2787 or Christian Chiropractors Association, 2550 Stover B-102, Fort Collins, CO, 80525.

David S. Jensen, DC, is a graduate of Parker College of Chiropractic. Dr. Dave has been in active practice for more than 16 years. He has worked with many different organizations ranging from professional football to Olympic athletes. His practice is in beautiful Aspen, Colorado, and he utilizes a multidisciplinary approach to healthcare. He is also working on a couple of other books that will be released soon and does public speaking engagements. You can reach Dr. Jensen by email at Drdave@winhealthinstitute.com or by phone at 970.279.4099 for a Balanced Approach to Health!

Leslie Kasanoff, DC, earned her Doctor of Chiropractic in 1989 from Western States Chiropractic College in Portland, Oregon. She practices part-time on the Central Coast of California. Dr. Kasanoff also devotes a significant amount of time to teaching people about healthy eating and whole food supplements through her

Juice Plus Virtual Franchise. Get more information at http://drlesliejuiceplus.com, http://coastchirowellness.com or contact her by email: kirokaz@sbcglobal.net.

Julie A. Kaufman, DC, CAC, completed the American Veterinary Chiropractic Association (AVCA) certification in 1990, earning the second Animal Chiropractic certification in the world. She owns a three-doctor integrative veterinary clinic, Animal Holistic Care Specialists of Wisconsin (AHCS). Dr. Kaufman is a 1989 graduate of Cleveland Chiropractic College. From 1989-1993, she was a regular lecturer for Options for Animals and AVCA. She has authored *Crossing the Rubicon: Celebrating the Human-Animal Bond in Life and Death* and *JointYoga for Animals: Strength, Flexibility, Balance.* Dr. Kaufman currently lectures worldwide on animal topics and also teaches a JointYoga certification course and an equine-assisted women's symposium on happiness and success. To learn more about AHCS and Dr. Kaufman's courses, call P: 608.655.1800, or visit W: www.JointYoga.com and www.ChiropracticforAnimals.net, E: arabequine@aol.com.

Tracy Kennedy-Shanks, DC, is a graduate of the Parker College of Chiropractic in Dallas, Texas. She may be contacted at the Kennedy Chiropractic Centre, 130 Russell Street, Toowoomba, Queensland, Australia 4350, P/F: 07.4639.1060, E: healthy@kennedychiro.com, W: www.kennedychiro.com. For a complimentary subscription to the Kennedy Chiropractic Centre newsletter, send your request to: newsletter@kennedychiro.com.

Peter W. Kfoury, DC (Doctor of Chiropractic), **DABCI** (Diplomate of the American Board of Chiropractic Internists), is in his 32nd year of practice. After graduating from Logan College of Chiropractic in 1978, Dr. Kfoury started a family practice in the Boston area where he remained for ten years. After relocating to Charleston, South Carolina, in 1989 (three months before Hurricane Hugo!) he decided to pursue the three-year Internist Diplomate program. His practice now includes a wide range of diagnostic and therapeutic options including multiple Chiropractic techniques, applied kinesiology, TBM (Total Body Modification), nutritional therapy, homeopathy, full lab workups, and laser therapy. Dr. Kfoury also enjoys playing music and softball and spending time with his most wonderful family.

Tedd Koren, DC, graduated from Sherman College of Chiropractic as class valedictorian. At Sherman, he was editor of the student newspaper. Today, he is the most well-read Doctor of Chiropractic in the world with over 50 million of his scientifically-referenced, patient education brochures in distribution. Dr. Koren founded and writes for Koren Publications, publisher of Chiropractic books, posters, office forms, stickers, and childhood vaccination materials: www.korenpublications.com. He produces a monthly newsletter for patients: www.patientnewsletter.com. Dr. Koren is the developer of Koren Specific Technique: www.korenspecifictechnique.com. Subscriptions to his doctor newsletter are free. E: tkoren1@aol.com, P: 215.699.7906.

Lori Krauss, DC, is a second-generation chiropractor who has been adjusted since birth. She has practiced Chiropractic in Colorado for 28 years, serving a large population of children and their families. She has served on several international mission trips to Brazil, Panama, and the Dominican Republic, and has served at a local residential treatment center for severely abused children. Dr.

Lori has been involved with Network Spinal Analysis, Dr. Donald Epstein's work, for 13 years and is on staff. She has three adult boys and a grandson, all of whom have been under Chiropractic care since birth. Dr. Lori can be reached at 970.310.9049 or sacredmission@comcast.net.

Gerald R. Kreitz, DC, is a 1987 graduate of the Texas Chiropractic College in Pasadena, Texas. His office is a family practice clinic focusing on chronic illnesses and long-term wellness. His emphasis is on structural correction and nutritional counseling. Dr. Kreitz is located at 16607 Blanco Road, Suite 1401, San Antonio, Texas 78232; P: 210.492.4433; E: grkreitzdc@yahoo.com.

Polly Camp Kreitz graduated in 1980 from Trinity University in San Antonio, Texas. She was the editor of *The Test Pad* and a contributing editor to *EEGink* when she worked for Automotive Research. Her work has also appeared in *Vantage Magazine*. Her short story, "A Plank Is the Deed to My Memories," was published in several inspirational anthologies. She has completed the first novel of a trilogy, *Magnolia Meadows*, with *Hollyhock Ridge* and *Salt Creek Falls* in progress. All three novels are set in Alabama.

Daniel F. Lavanga, DC, has been a practicing chiropractor for more than 22 years and is an author, speaker, and executive coach. He is the president of the Lavanga Group, a corporate consultancy specializing in personal and professional leadership and health management, executive coaching, and people process development. He operates a life and health training program for physicians, others desirous of a coaching career, and a personal fitness certification program for fitness instructors. His book, *The Law Of Sevens*, is a fitness program for the mind. The Lavanga Group, 112 E. Pennsylvania Boulevard, Feasterville, PA 19053, 215-364-1112, or at www.thelavangagroup.com.

Carol Le Blanc, DC, chose Chiropractic as a second career following a skiing accident and subsequent Chiropractic care. She graduated from Cleveland Chiropractic College-Los Angeles in1985. Using her love of communication, teaching skills, and motivation, she spoke at Parker Seminars on self-discovery, health, and networking. Awarded Woman Chiropractor of the Year PSPS 1991-92 and Doctor of the Year-1996, she was instrumental in the formation of the World Congress of Women Chiropractors. She continues her family practice of 24 years specializing in Activator technique with a focus on lifetime wellness care. Her practice is located at 20301 SW Acacia Street, Suite 150, Newport Beach, California, 949.645.9050.

Leigh Frisbee Lenz, DC, CVCP, is a graduate of Parker College of Chiropractic in Dallas, Texas, and has completed her post-graduate Animal Chiropractic certification. She is a graduate of the University of Mississippi where she played soccer for four years. She enjoys flying, sports, outdoor activities, and helping others reach their optimal health potential through lifestyle changes and Chiropractic. She is married to Dr. Scott R. Lenz, a successful chiropractor and race car driver, and has two healthy and busy boys, Bradley and Brandon. For more information about Dr. Leigh's practice, please visit www.lenzchiropractic.com or call 541.826.6800.

Rose Lepien, DC, received her Associates Degree in Science from Cameron University in Lawton, Oklahoma, and her Doctorate of Chiropractic degree from the Parker College of Chiropractic in Dallas, Texas, in 1991. A

Chiropractic veteran of 37 years, she has given back to her profession through leadership in the Parker College Alumni Association, Parker Seminars, the World Congress of Women Chiropractors, and has served ten years on the Board of Trustees of Parker College of Chiropractic, and four years as Chairman of the Board. She continues to bloom where she is planted, treating patients and touching lives at the Aaragon Chiropractic Clinic in Lawton, Oklahoma. E: drrose@fidnet.com, W: www.aaragonchiropractic.com, or P: 580.353.6776.

Anastasia Line is a reformed "non-believer" in Chiropractic who now works with well-known Family Wellness Chiropractor and international lecturer, Dr. Claudia Anrig, in the mentoring of other like-minded Doctors of Chiropractic. As the Generations Liaison, Anastasia supports Dr. Anrig as she helps other chiropractors reach the women in their community who, typically, are the healthcare decision makers for their families. Working with Dr. Anrig, Anastasia has many opportunities to promote the wellness message and be an advocate for family wellness Chiropractic care. To learn more about children and Chiropractic visit www.icpa4kids.org or email Anastasia directly at anastasialine@prodigy.net.

Brandi MacDonald has led large, multi-disciplinary teams in support of women, children, and families living in poverty. During this period, she was touched by the healing power of Chiropractic and changed her career. Today, an advocate of wellness, wife of a chiropractor, and motivating leader, she owns True Concepts Inc. providing consulting and professional speaking services to the Chiropractic profession and women's wellness groups. You may contact Brandi at P: 780.439.3444; E: info@brandimacdonald.com; W: www.brandimacdonald.com; or Southside Chiropractic and Health Centre; W: www.edmontonchirosouthside.com; .

Christie MacDonald, DC, graduated from the Canadian Memorial Chiropractic College in 1997 and completed her Animal Chiropractic certification at The Healing Oasis Wellness Centre of Canada in 2007. Whitemud Crossing Chiropractors is located at 141, 4211 106th Street, Edmonton, Alberta, Canada 56J 6P3; E: info@whitemudcrossingchiropractors.com; P: 780.430.7549; F: 780.430.7453; W: www.whitemudcrossingchiropractors.com. Kennedy Chiropractic Centre newsletter, send your request to: newsletter@kennedychiro.com.

Catherine Maloof, DC, graduated from the Los Angeles College of Chiropractic in 1988. For more than twenty years, she has been in private practice in Mission Viejo, California, specializing in Family Health Care, Nutritional Therapy, Sports Injuries, and taking people's health to the next level. Dr. Maloof is a speaker and author as well and has made a profound difference through her empowering library of learning materials including books, DVDs and CDs. You may find additional information on her website, www.drmaloof.com, and sign up for her free online newsletter. She can be reached at 949.581.6543 or drmaloof@aol.com.

Cody J. Masek, DC, graduated from the College of Chiropractic at Minnesota's Northwestern Health Sciences University in 2003. His office is a family practice clinic focusing on long-term wellness. Complete Health Chiropractic welcomes new patients and is located at 27420 Jefferson Avenue, Suite 104A, Temecula, CA 92590; P: 951.693.5629; F: 951.693.4197; E: drcodymasek@yahoo.com; W: www.completehealthtemecula.com.

David Neubauer, DC, is a 1983 graduate of Northwestern Health Sciences

University. After years of small town practice in rural Minnesota (Bird Island), he now consults and trains for HealthSource Chiropractic and Progressive Rehab, a national Chiropractic franchise. He lectures throughout the United States, Canada and South America on personal development, TEAM building and systems of operation in business. His greatest personal joy comes from his marriage to his beautiful wife, Carrie, and his three children, Cole, Ross, and Anne—all now young adults. You may contact Dr. David Neubauer @ E: dneubauer@healthsourcechiro.com, P: 952.937.0127, or 8603 Lake Riley Drive, Chanhassen, MN 55317.

Erik H. Norslien, DC, is a 1995 graduate of Palmer College of Chiropractic in Davenport, Iowa. He has practiced in Lewistown, Montana, since 1999. Dedicated to delivering health and wellness, Dr. Norslien utilizes a multitude of Chiropractic techniques and has spent countless hours studying the best approaches for helping his patients. Dr. Norslien's office is located at 204 NE Main Street, Lewistown, MT 59457, P: 406.528.7201.

Jeanne Ohm, DC, has practiced family wellness care since 1981 with her husband, Dr. Tom. They have six children who were all born at home and are living the Chiropractic family wellness lifestyle. Dr. Ohm is an instructor, author, and innovator. Her passions are training DCs with specific techniques for care in pregnancy, birth and infancy, forming national alliances for chiropractors with like-minded perinatal practitioners, empowering mothers to make informed choices, and offering pertinent patient educational materials.

Richard Parenti, DC, RMA, graduated from New York Chiropractic College in 1996. As a certified Educator and a Registered Medical Assistant, he serves as the Medical Program Director of an Associate Degree Medical Assisting program in North Carolina. In 2008, Dr. Parenti started the non-profit organization, Dry Kid Academy, that teaches kids how to stay dry in their bed at night. He currently serves as the Executive Director of the organization and has helped kids throughout the United States. Dr. Parenti has a part-time Chiropractic practice and has coined himself as the "un-Chiropractor" because of his unusual background and experience as well as his unique contribution to the Chiropractic profession. For information about bedwetting, visit Dry Kid Academy online at: www.drykid.org.

Bradley R. Pennington, DC, graduated from Cleveland Chiropractic College of Kansas City, Missouri, in 1990. Since then, he has provided Chiropractic adjustments in 6 countries on 3 continents, operated clinics for large Chiropractic chains, been a provider in various wellness facilities, and has owned and operated 3 businesses including a day spa in the Vail valley. His Chiropractic "career" began when he was 10 years old and experienced firsthand the miracles of Chiropractic care for himself in a small rural Alaskan town. He currently resides and practices in Denver, Colorado, and is also available to travel and provide Chiropractic care for distinguished, private clientele. You may contact Dr. Pennington at E: drbrad@bradpennington.com, W: www.bradpennington.com, P: 970.688.0097, 1115 Broadway, Suite 109, Denver CO 80203.

Steven J. Pollack, DC, is a graduate of Life Chiropractic College and Director of Pollack Health and Wellness Center, Beachwood, New Jersey. The author of two books, *Ask the Chiropractor I* and *II*, Dr. Pollack has written over 700 self-help columns on wellness for a wide variety of newspapers and other periodicals. Dr. Pollack has passionately practiced Chiropractic for 29 years, is a founding member of the Council of Chiropractic Pediatrics and International Chiropractic Pediatric Association and a member of the Chiropractic Knights of the Round Table. Dr. Pollack lives with his wife, Patricia, and their four children along the Jersey Shore.

Ray Pope, DC, is a graduate of Sherman College of Chiropractic in Spartanburg, South Carolina. He has enjoyed a vital practice on Camano Island in Washington State since 1985. He completed postgraduate studies under the late I. N. Toftness, DC, PhC, and has continued to earn specialized certifications from NeuroMechanical Systems, Texas Chiropractic College, and Kinesio Tapping Association International. The Pope's have five adult children and enjoy living fully in the Northwest as well as serving on short-term mission teams to Mexico. He can be reached at drpope@openthegift.org.

Tom Potisk, DC, is a graduate of Palmer College of Chiropractic. He is known worldwide as The "Down-to-Earth" doctor because of his holistic lifestyle and easygoing teaching ability. After 25 years of operating a busy, multi-doctor family practice, he is now a public speaker advocating holistic health—especially Chiropractic care. His new books, *Whole Health Healing: The Budget Friendly Natural Wellness Bible for All Ages* and *Reclaim the Joy of Practice: An Advanced Guide for Advancing Doctors*, are available on his website at www.thedowntoearthdoctor.com. Contact Dr. Tom Potisk at 262.835.1767 or Email: tpotisk@aol.com.

James P. Powell, DC, graduated from National College of Chiropractic in 1970 and is celebrating 40 years in practice. He practices with son James D. Powell, DC, sons-in-law Walter B. Null, DC, Daniel P. Smith, DC, and youngest son, Robert D. Powell, ND. Dr. Powell has served as District II representative of the FCLB. He served eight years on the Ohio Chiropractic Board and four years as its President. He is also a member of the Board of Trustees of the New York Chiropractic College. He lives in Canton, Ohio, with his wife of 44 years, Donna. They have four adult children and thirteen grandchildren. Dr. Powell currently serves as a consultant to Standard Process.

Jeffrey Ptak, DC, graduated with honors from the Los Angeles College of Chiropractic. He is the owner of Ptak Wellness in West Los Angeles, California, and has been in private practice for 25 years. As a founding member of CREW—Chiropractors Restoring Energy Worldwide, Dr. Ptak has made an impact on natural health and healing on a global level through lectures, workshops, and mission trips to Cuba, Panama, and other locations. Dr. Ptak is currently enrolled in the MA program in Spiritual Psychology at the University of Santa Monica in Santa Monica, California, and continues to deepen his focus on the relationship between consciousness, healing, and spirituality. You may reach Dr. Ptak at W: www.ptakchiropractic.com or P: 310.473.7991.

Nima Rahmany, DC, is a 2001 graduate of the Canadian Memorial Chiropractic College in Toronto. Previously, he attended the University of British Columbia's Kinesiology program. After associating for almost six years, he is currently the owner of one of the largest multi-disciplinary, alternative healing centers in the greater Vancouver area—with fourteen practitioners and seven staff—serving thousands of clients monthly. Westgate Wellness Centre has now turned into a teaching center where clients not only come to get well, but learn how to empower their lives in all areas to *stay* well physically, emotionally, and relationally, and to have more fulfilling lives. To contact Dr. Nima, please visit his website and blog, www.DrNima.com. P: 604.465.HAND.

William C. Remling, DC, FICA, graduated from the Chiropractic Institute of New York in 1963. He returned to his alma mater to teach for several years while in private practice in Glendale, New York. He served his last ten years in New York as the Founder and Executive Director for the New York Chiropractic Council. Bill devoted his time and energy to getting Insurance Equality legislation passed in New York State against heavy odds. A teacher, writer, and lecturer in Chiropractic, health and wellness, "Bill" is now living in Surprise, Arizona with his wife, Kathy. He can be reached at chirobill@aol.com.

Dorrin B. Rosenfeld, DC, graduated from Life Chiropractic College-West in 1992. She previously earned her BA from Amherst College in 1985 and amassed her real-life experience over the next three years in the Peace Corps in Belize and in the Greenery, a head-injury rehabilitation center in Massachusetts. She currently specializes in Blair Upper Cervical Chiropractic and concentrates on Patient Neurology and its far-reaching effects. She practices at 326 De Anza Drive in Vallejo, CA 94589. E: drdim@comcast.net, P: 707.557.5471, W: www.StateoftheArtChiro.com and www.MiracleChiro.com.

Sandi Rosier, LMT, MTI, is a Licensed Massage Therapist and Massage Therapy Instructor. She earned her LMT in 2004 at the Texas Massage Institute in Ft. Worth. Sandi's primary motivation in pursuing this career was to help her young daughter, Teddi, cope with epileptic seizures. Sandi discovered that massage therapy and Chiropractic—working together—can do wonders in restoring and maintaining spinal health. Sandi's Body Spa is located in Keller, Texas, and about 25 percent of her clients are referrals from chiropractors. It gives her enormous satisfaction to be a part of the natural healthcare profession. You may reach Sandi at 817.729.3055.

Eric G. Russell, DC, is a 1996 graduate of Palmer College of Chiropractic. Pursuing his passion of Chiropractic philosophy, Dr. Russell is an Associate Professor at Parker College of Chiropractic while maintaining a busy private practice. Because of his love for the Chiropractic profession, he is an international speaker, author, and teacher. Dr. Russell lives in Commerce, Texas, with his wonderful wife, Yvonne Villanueava-Russell, PhD, and their son, Blake. You may email Dr. Russell at erussell@parkercc.edu.

Gregory R. Salmond, DC, is a 1981 graduate of Life University. After experiencing many personal health benefits as a child and being inspired by his personal chiropractor, the late Bruce Merritt, DC, and family, Dr. Salmond runs a Health and Wellness Chiropractic center located at 272 Route 206, Suite 212, Flanders, NJ 07836. His emphasis is on the health benefits that Chiropractic has to offer both young and old alike. P: 973.927.8522, F: 973.927.9888, E: greg.salmond@gmail.com, W: www.gmrcreations.com/Salmond.

Terry Schroeder, DC, is a graduate of Palmer College of Chiropractic West in San Jose, California. He and his wife, Lori Schroeder, DC, have owned and run a family-oriented practice for the past 23 years in Westlake Village, California. Dr. Schroeder is America's only four-time Olympian in the sport of water polo. He is a two-time silver medalist as an athlete and is presently the Head Coach for Team USA. His team won a silver medal in Beijing in 2008 and is aiming for gold in London in 2012. He may be contacted at Schroeder Center for Healthy Living, 31225 La Baya Drive, Suite 206, Westlake Village, CA 91361. P: 818.889.5572, F: 818. 889.7368, E: tschroeder@usawaterpolo.org or W: www.schroederhealthyliving.com.

James Sigafoose, DC, a 1959 graduate of National College of Chiropractic, is recognized worldwide for his inspirational Chiropractic philosophy and motivational skills. As a Team Teacher for Parker Seminars since 1995 and a presenter at Dynamic Essentials (D.E.) for over 25 years, Dr. Sigafoose has spoken to audiences worldwide including Europe, Canada, USA, Japan, and Australia. He was one of 18 chiropractors to attend the Good Will Games in Moscow, one of 20 to participate in the Haiti mission, and one of 25 in the Panama mission. He is the author of *Good Medicine* as well as a variety of Chiropractic educational audio and video tapes.

David Singer, DC, received his undergraduate degree from Rutgers University, his MS degree in nutrition from the University of Bridgeport, and his doctorate from the New York College of Chiropractic in 1972. Dr. Singer built one of the largest practices in the world and then founded his own consulting company in 1981 that has twice won the prestigious *Inc.* magazine's Top 100 Fastest Growing Companies Award. He is currently on the advisory board of the ACA's Legal Action Fund, Chiropractic Summit and both *In Practice* magazine and *The American Chiropractor*. He received the "Person of the Year Award" from *Chiropractic Economics*. Dr. Singer is considered one of the most inspiring, humorous, and articulate speakers in Chiropractic. To attend one of his seminars or teleconferences, please call 800.326.1797.

Frank Sovinsky, DC, is a graduate of Palmer College of Chiropractic. As the founder and CEO of DC Mentors, he is transforming the lives of chiropractors and their patients worldwide. He is the co-author of *The E-Myth Chiropractor* and author of *Life the Manual*. His passion and genius for understanding human behavior and motivation makes him a popular speaker and mentor. To contact Dr. Sovinsky, you may email him at info@dcmentors.com or visit his website and blog at www.dcmentors.com .

Kirtland J. Speaks, DC, is a 1994 graduate of Logan College of Chiropractic. He and his wife, Lisa, own Expressions Chiropractic and Rehab, P.A. located in Cedar Hill and North Richland Hills, Texas. He has been practicing for over 15 years, and is an adjunct professor for Parker College. He is very involved in community leadership and organizations and is the team doctor for a local high school. Lisa works at Parker College of Chiropractic and is a team teacher for Parker Seminars. Both are amazed at the miracles they see through Chiropractic and hope that they can reach more people through education and involvement. Phone: 972.291.4455. You can visit Dr. Speaks on his website at www.expressionschiropractic.com.

David H. Spear, PhD, DC, earned a PhD in biological chemistry from the University of California Los Angeles, prior to receiving his Doctor of Chiropractic degree in 2000 from Life Chiropractic College West. Dr. Spear and his wife, Melody Spear, DC, have a family wellness practice in Eugene, Oregon. Their office specializes in the care of children and expectant mothers. Dr. Spear may be contacted at P: 541.687.7775, E: David@body-of-light.com and W: www.body-of-light.com.

Michael Staffen DC, is a graduate of Canadian Memorial Chiropractic College in Toronto. He believes in giving back both to his profession and his community. Dr. Staffen is president of the Sudbury Chiropractic Society, organizes Chiropractic seminars, serves as Peer Evaluator for CCO, and mentors students. As part of his community involvement, he is a founding member and president of the Joe MacDonald Youth Football League, coaches football, and is an active member of the Rotary Club of Sudbury Sunrisers. Dr Staffen's family, wife, Darlene, and four children, epitomize the Chiropractic Lifestyle. He can be contacted at drmikestaffen@sympatico.ca.

Barbara V. Thomas, DC, was a Newburgh, New York, Dominican nun from 1958-1973. She graduated from the Columbia Institute of Chiropractic at New York City College in 1973. Dr. Thomas is married to Barney Thomas who also graduated from CIC. Both Barbara and Barney are ordained ministers in the Spiritualist Church. They have a son, Martin R., who lives in the Bronx, New York. Barbara practices at 1568 Route 80 in Guilford, Connecticut. P: 203.457.1078. E: Chirobvt@yahoo.com. W: www.bthomaschiropractic.com.

John G. Watson, DC, graduated from Palmer College of Chiropractic in 1983 at the age of 42, with ten children in tow. He had turned down a principalship in an elementary school to pursue a career in Chiropractic and probably holds the record for—if not the oldest student—then at least the graduate with the most children to support. Dr. Watson set up practice in Hendersonville, North Carolina, where he retired in 2007 with 13 children and 43 grandchildren. You can tell he loves little children, as his story testifies. Dr. Watson was invited to share his account at the Palmer College of Chiropractic Homecoming in May, 2006.

William C. Werner, DC, earned a BSc at the University of Toronto in 1970 and graduated from Canadian Memorial Chiropractic College in Toronto in 1974. He has enjoyed a private family practice for 36 years, serving the rural and growing industrial community located on the north shore of Lake Erie in southern Ontario. You may contact Dr. Werner at Werner Chiropractic Office, 12 Alma Street S, Hagersville, Ontario N0A 1H0, Canada. P: 905.768.5834, F: 905.768.1721, E: wernerchiro@mountaincable.net.

Elisabeth Wiebe earned a Bachelor of Sacred Music degree from FaithWay Baptist College of Canada after which she married the love of her life, David. She is a full-time mom of three wonderful children. Her second daughter, Julia, has a rare chromosome disorder. Through Julia's health difficulties, Elisabeth learned about the importance of Chiropractic care and is now a firm believer that the first line of defense for the human body is a Chiropractic adjustment. Presently, she ministers alongside her husband, pastor of Toronto's New Life Baptist Church.

She is thankful to God for all His blessings, and realizes that all healing comes from Him. E: liz.wiebe@gmail.com, W: www.considernewlife.org.

T. D. Wilson, DC, is a proud graduate of Parker College of Chiropractic. Dr. Wilson is a Wellness Entrepreneur at heart. He is a family wellness chiropractor who owns and operates a whole wellness center that has five doctors, five massage therapists, a counselor, a Creating Wellness™ Center, and a complete nutrition store that serves organic smoothies, coffee, and tea. Dr. Wilson also speaks nationally to the profession and the public to further the Chiropractic message. Dr. Wilson shares his life with his loving wife Amy and their five children in Lubbock, Texas. He can be reached through the office website at www.CreateYourWellness.com.

Curry Y. L. Wong, DC, CACCP, is a graduate of the Life Chiropractic College West. She is certified by the Academy of Family Practice and is Webster Technique Certified. Dr. Wong's post-graduate study qualifies her to specialize in Chiropractic for pediatrics, expectant mothers, and female care. She is a licensed chiropractor with Chiropractors Council of the Hong Kong and is a member of International Chiropractic Pediatric Association, International Chiropractors Association, and Chiropractic Doctors' Association of Hong Kong. She may be contacted at LGS International Chiropractic, 1 Coleman Street #04-26, The Adelphi, Singapore 179803, Singapore. P: 65.6338.7470, E: drcwong@lgsic.com, W: www.lgsic.com.

Joshua J. Wood, 28 years of age, has a motto: "Twice Born." His "first life" covered the interval from birth until his accident on June 25, 2000, when he crashed on an asphalt road while attempting a snowboard jump. Diagnosed as a complete quadriplegic, he suffered a crushed spinal cord with less than 10% bodily function. Although his medical prognosis was grim, his chiropractor, Dr. Simon Floreani, has spent the last ten years—Josh's "second life"— proving the medical profession wrong. Josh walks without any modifications, rides a motor bike, drives a car, snowboards, and runs a web-based business at www.blackmoneyclothing.com.

Trevor Van Wyk, DC, is a graduate of Logan College of Chiropractic in Chesterfield, Missouri. A third-generation chiropractor, Dr. Van Wyk practices with his father, Dr. Chris Van Wyk, at Van Wyk Family Chiropractic Center in Littleton, Colorado. In addition to Chiropractic practice, Dr. Van Wyk is an author, lecturer, and business and marketing consultant. Dr. Van Wyk and his wife, Angie, are busy raising three wonderful boys and enjoy spending time with their family and friends. To contact Dr. Trevor Van Wyk, call his office at 303-794-8754.

Christine B. Zack, CLTC, is a Certified Long Term Care professional and Reiki Master in Eugene, Oregon. She currently owns Silver Solutions, a Retirement and Health Care consultancy. She began study with her grandfather, a professional healer, in the '50s and works with seniors in healthcare and retirement planning. She assists her clients, in a loving way, to transition the next phase of life ensuring that all areas of health, income, LTC, legacy planning and final wishes are handled. Her medical intuition leads her to push through conventional treatments for her clients by providing emotional support and educational resources. E: christinebzack@comcast.net.

Permissions Acknowledgments

"I Love You, Mommy!" was originally published in *Pathways to Family Wellness Magazine* in June 2005 by the International Chiropractic Pediatric Association, Media, Pennsylvania, under the title, "Zachary's Story," and is reprinted here in adapted form with permission from Susan Boerchers. © 2005, 2010 Susan Boerchers.

"A Life-Changing Event" was originally published in *Pathways to Family Wellness Magazine* in March 2005 by the International Chiropractic Pediatric Association, Media, Pennsylvania, under the title, "Eric's Story," and is reprinted here in adapted form with permission from Christine B. Zack, CLTC. © 2005, 2010 Christine B. Zack.

"Teddi's New 'Favorite Thing to Do' " was originally published in *Pathways to Family Wellness Magazine* in January 2010 by the International Chiropractic Pediatric Association, Media, Pennsylvania, under the title, "Teddi's Story," and is reprinted here in adapted form with permission from Sandi Rosier, LMT, MTI. © 2010 Sandi Rosier.

"How I Avoided Neck Surgery" was originally published on the website, www.demosschiropractic.com, Newport Beach, California, and is reprinted here in adapted form with permission from Bill DeMoss, DC. © 2010 Bill DeMoss.

"Good Tidings from Singapore" was originally published on the website, www.lgsic.com, Singapore, under the title, "Testimonial 1," and is reprinted here in adapted form with permission from Curry Wong, DC. © 2007-2010 LGS International Chiropractic.

"No More Migraines!" was originally published on www.bradpennington.com, Denver, Colorado, under the title, "Testimonial," and is reprinted here in adapted form with permission from Brad Pennington, DC. © 2010 Denver Chiropractic.

"Firefighter: Every Kid's Dream" was originally published on the website, www.caputochiropracticri.com, Cranston, Rhode Island, under the title, "Chiropractic Testimonials: David Dinobile," and is reprinted here in adapted form with permission from Edward Caputo, DC and Judith Gallagher, DC. © 2003 caputochiropracticri.com.